CONTENTS

Dedication 1
Author's Note 2
About the Author 3
Connect With Me 5
Chapter 1: Breaking the Spell 6
Chapter 2: The System Isn't Sick 18
Chapter 3: The Poison in the Products 41
Chapter 4: The Body Remembers 65
Chapter 5: Rewilding the Feminine 82
Chapter 6: The Truth About Healing 97
Chapter 7: Detoxing the Mind, Spirit & Soul 115
Chapter 8: Building a Life That Heals You 133
Chapter 9: Raising the Next Generation Free 151
Chapter 10: Sovereignty as a Lifestyle 165
Chapter 11: The Separation Myth 178
Chapter 12: The War on the Body 199
Chapter 13: Addicted to Healing 218
Aftercare 233
Acknowledgements 236
Resources 237
Glossary 238

DEDICATION

To the wild ones who never stopped seeking, the wounded ones who dared to heal, and the waking ones who chose to remember.

This is for you.

And to my children, may you always trust your truth, walk your own path, and know that magic runs through your veins.

Author's Note

There was a time I believed healing meant becoming someone else. More acceptable. More functional. More... quiet.

But healing was never about erasing who I was. It was about remembering who I had always been.

This book is the sacred map I never had for those ready to dismantle, decode, and rise out of the matrix of self-abandonment. Written not just from lived experience, but through years of spiritual study, soul reclamation, and academic research in the field of metaphysical sciences.

May it meet you in your softness, your fire, your rage, and your return. You don't need fixing. You need freedom.

And you don't have to earn that. It's already yours.

With reverence and rebellion,
Dr. Hannah Strange, PhD
Metaphysical Sciences

About the Author

Dr. Hannah Strange, PhD is a metaphysical scientist, holistic health practitioner, spiritual mentor, and founder of The Strange Apothecary. A modern day alchemist with roots in rebellion, Hannah weaves together ancient wisdom, intuitive medicine, and soul science to support others on their path of radical healing and self-liberation.

She holds a PhD in Metaphysical Sciences and has spent her life in devotion to healing, both her own and that of others. Her work is both lived and learned, grounded in personal experience, trauma informed care, and spiritual sovereignty.

She is the host of The Sacred Code Podcast, creator of The Sacred Portal, and a fierce advocate for living a sacred life outside the systems that were never built for us.

Hannah lives in the UK with her magical, neurodivergent family, where she blends apothecary work, homeschooling, tree planting, and truth-telling into an enchanted life of rebellion and reverence.

The Sacred Rebellion: A healing revolution for the wild, the wounded, and the waking.
© 2025 Hannah Strange, PhD
All rights reserved.

No part of this publication may be reproduced, stored in a retrieval system, or transmitted in any form or by any means, electronic, mechanical, photocopying, recording, or otherwise without prior written permission from the author.

This book is a work of nonfiction based on personal experience, professional insight, and academic research in the field of metaphysical sciences. While every effort has been made to ensure accuracy, this book is not a substitute for medical advice. Readers are encouraged to consult qualified professionals where needed.

First edition, 2025
Printed in the United Kingdom

Connect With Me

Let's stay in rebellion together.

Website: strangeapothecary.co.uk
Instagram: @strangeapothecary
Podcast: The Sacred Code (available on Spotify, Apple, and all major platforms).
Work With Me: Join The Sacred Portal or explore The Sacred Forest Membership on my website strangeapothecary.co.uk
Email: contact@strangeapothecary.co.uk

Tag me when you read, underline, highlight, cry, or scream YES while reading, this is your rebellion too.

CHAPTER 1

Breaking the Spell

You were never meant to just survive, you were built to thrive.

There's a moment in every sacred rebellion where the veil begins to thin. It doesn't come with sirens. No red flags. No dramatic music or grand announcements. Just a quiet, gnawing discomfort. A single thought that won't leave you alone:

"This can't be it."

Maybe it comes while you're sitting in the waiting room at your GP for the third time that month. Maybe it slips in as you open another bottle of multicoloured tablets lined up next to your child's cereal box. Maybe it shows up in the middle of the night, when the kids are asleep, and you're sitting in the bathroom wondering why your body still doesn't feel like home after all this time.

You brush it off. At first. Because that's what we've been trained to do, override the warning signs. Push through. Numb out. Take the pill. Be grateful.

But something deep in your bones keeps whispering: "This isn't right. You were meant for more than this." That whisper is sacred. That whisper is the beginning. And once you hear it, the spell begins to crack.

We Were Born Into the Fog

Before you could name your body parts or speak your truth, you were absorbing the world around you. You were told how to sit, how to speak, how to behave. What to eat, when to sleep, when to ask for permission to simply feel. And over time, you became fluent in a language that told you your power wasn't yours to hold.

You were taught:

That sickness was inevitable.
That the doctor always knows best.
That symptoms are mistakes to be silenced.
That your body is a ticking time bomb.
That your intuition is irrational.
That healing is external, complicated, and definitely not free.

From the moment we entered this world, we were immersed in a culture of silent obedience disguised as wellness. We were given over-the-counter medicine instead of being taught how to feel into discomfort. We were told to calm down instead of being asked what do you need? We were rewarded for ignoring our bodies and punished for listening to them.

And we called it normal.

The "Good Girl" Spell

For many women, the conditioning goes deeper.

We were raised to be good. To be easy. To be small.
To not question authority. To not inconvenience others.
To say "I'm fine" when we were breaking inside.
To smile when we were dismissed, to stay silent when we were ignored.

We were taught that being "difficult" meant being less lovable. That being "emotional" meant being irrational. That being intuitive, sensitive, reactive, overwhelmed, meant we were the problem.

So, we internalised it. We turned against our own bodies.
We numbed with sugar, caffeine, scrolling, shopping, compliance.
We dieted away our instincts. We medicated away our symptoms.

We trained ourselves to be palatable, while our spirit rotted quietly under the surface.

This is the spell. And it's not your fault. But it is your time to break it.

The Wake-Up Call (And Why It Often Looks Like Chaos)

Most of us didn't wake up in a gentle yoga flow with green juice in hand. We woke up when our health collapsed. When a diagnosis shook our foundation. When our children got sick and no one could explain why. When our body stopped cooperating. When our anxiety became unbearable. When our sixth GP appointment in six months left us with nothing but another prescription and an empty feeling in our gut.

The body is wise.
She will whisper… then nudge… then shout.

Symptoms aren't punishments. They are sacred messengers.
They are your body begging you to stop ignoring her.

What you thought was the problem, your fatigue, your gut issues, your hormonal chaos, was actually the portal.
You weren't being broken. You were being invited.

The Nervous System Spell

You can't heal what you're too numb to feel. And most of us are numb. Not because we're broken, but because we're biologically overwhelmed.

Your nervous system was never designed for this much input, this much pressure, this much noise. We were meant to rise with the sun, move our bodies gently, tend to the land, connect in community, and rest when needed.

Instead?

We're bombarded with toxins, deadlines, trauma, stimulants, screens, and endless noise. We run on caffeine and cortisol. We're expected to be mothers, bosses, lovers, healers, housekeepers, CEOs and calm, functioning humans, without faltering.

And when our nervous systems scream "enough", we're told we're being dramatic. When our bodies collapse, there's a pill for that. When our emotions erupt, there's therapy, medication, or a label to silence it.

But what if your overwhelm was a sacred alarm? What if your dysregulation was your body saying: "You're not supposed to live like this."

We weren't built for endless productivity. We were built for presence. For cycles. For stillness. For joy.

The nervous system spell tells us to cope, manage, suppress. The rebellion says: Regulate, rest, reclaim.

The Sacred Grief

Waking up doesn't feel empowering at first. It feels devastating.

There's grief in awakening, deep, guttural, unspoken grief.

You grieve the version of you who trusted all the wrong things. You grieve the time lost to sickness. You grieve the years your child suffered because you didn't know better. You grieve the person you had to become just to survive.

And underneath that grief... comes rage.

Rage at the industries that lied. Rage at the schools that never taught you how to listen to your body. Rage at the doctors who dismissed you. Rage at the inner critic who still whispers that you're too much.

Let that grief come. Let that rage rise. You are not too sensitive, you are finally sensing. You are not crazy, you are seeing clearly.

Grieve what needs grieving. Burn what needs burning. And then… rise from the ashes.

Why Perfection Is a Cage

Here's a trap no one warns you about: once you begin to awaken, you'll feel the pull to get it "right."

You'll want to clean your diet, ditch every chemical, regulate your nervous system, meditate daily, and heal every trauma… by Tuesday.

You'll find yourself obsessing over ingredient labels and blaming yourself for every slip-up. You'll cry because you forgot to take your supplements. You'll beat yourself up for getting sick, even when you've "done all the things."

That's not healing. That's control disguised as consciousness.

You don't have to be perfect to be powerful.
You don't have to do it all at once.
You don't have to be fully healed to start helping others.

Your journey is sacred because it's real.
Not because it's flawless.

You are allowed to be messy.
You are allowed to be in progress.
You are allowed to be both wounded and wise.

The spell of perfection is just another distraction from your sovereignty.

And you, wild one, were never here to perform, you were here to embody.

Reclaiming Sovereignty

Once you realise the spell exists, there's no unseeing it. You begin to notice things others still call normal:

The fragrance aisle giving you a headache.
The school lunch menu making your skin crawl.
The way people roll their eyes when you ask about ingredients.
The exhaustion hidden behind "I'm fine."
The dependency disguised as health care.

And while others keep marching in rhythm to the system's song, you begin to step out of time. You begin to remember your own beat. You begin to reclaim choice.

Sovereignty doesn't mean you know everything. It means you know yourself.

It means you get to say:

"I need time to think before I say yes."
"I'm not comfortable with that treatment."
"I'll try a natural approach first."
"I'm allowed to trust my gut over a Google search."
"My healing journey doesn't have to look like anyone else's."

You're not being stubborn.
You're not being difficult.
You're not being woo.

You are reclaiming the one thing the system relies on you never owning. Your own power.

The Wild Woman Returns

There is a part of you that was never spellbound. She is ancient. Untameable. Alive.
She is barefoot in the forest, singing to the wind.
She is stirring herbs by candlelight.
She is tattooed in dirt and moonlight.
She is you, beneath the layers.
You, before the silence.
You, before the system.
She is your inner wild woman.
And she is coming home.

You may feel her in moments:

When you instinctively reach for a tincture instead of a tablet.
When your body says no before your mouth catches up.
When you cry for no reason and then feel... relief.
When you look in the mirror and see yourself again.

She is not here to be convenient.
She is not here to be small.
She is not here to be saved.

She is your fiercest ally.
She is your inner healer.
And she is ready to rise.

Mini Ritual: Spellbreaker's Breath

You'll need: Just your body.

1. Find a quiet place. Sit or stand with your feet firmly rooted.
2. Close your eyes. Inhale through your nose for four counts.
3. Hold your breath for four.
4. Exhale slowly through your mouth for six.
5. Repeat this cycle three times.

Place your hand on your heart. Then on your womb, or belly.

And say aloud:

*"I release the lies I was raised to believe.
I am not broken. I was built for truth.
I trust the whispers of my body.
I honour the grief that brought me here.
And I now reclaim the power I was taught to fear.
This is my sacred rebellion. And I'm just getting started."*

Let the words land.
Let your breath settle.
Let your spine remember.

Sacred Journal Prompts

What parts of myself have I hidden to be acceptable or convenient?
Where am I still performing healing, instead of embodying it?
What does it feel like to honour the part of me that always knew something wasn't right?
What messages has my body been sending me that I've ignored?
What one thing can I do today that supports my sovereignty?

The Spell is Breaking

You made it here.

To the page where everything begins to shift. To the first page of a new language, one written in intuition, nature, remembrance, and power. You don't need to know what comes next. You just need to keep walking.

Because this isn't just a book. It's a portal you have stepped through and what lies ahead is nothing less than a return to yourself.

Chapter 2

The System Isn't Sick, It's Designed That Way

You've begun to awaken. You're noticing things you never questioned before. You're asking the hard questions, peeling back the layers, seeing through the marketing, the manipulation, the fear-based language.

And you're probably wondering:

How did we get here?
How did we become so disconnected from the natural way of living, healing, and knowing?
Why are we only now realising we've been kept sick, dependent, and exhausted, on purpose?

This isn't just about your personal healing anymore.
This is about the system that benefits from your suppression.

It is time to say it out loud:

The healthcare system we were raised to trust was not built for healing. It was built for profit. It was built for control. It was built for quiet compliance.

And once you see that truth, you stop expecting that system to hand you your wellness.

The Illusion of Care

Let's begin with the most sacred betrayal of all, the illusion that the system is here to take care of you.

From childhood, we're fed the narrative that:

The doctor knows best.
Pills are the answer.
Symptoms are problems.
Prevention means screening, not lifestyle.
Natural healing is "alternative," risky, or unscientific.

You go in with symptoms, fatigue, heavy periods, gut pain, mood swings, and leave with a prescription or a dismissal. If you're lucky, maybe a leaflet. There is rarely curiosity. Rarely time. Rarely a moment spent asking, "What is your body trying to tell you?"

We're taught that the doctor is the authority, and we are simply bodies to be diagnosed and managed.

But here's the truth they don't want you to remember:

Your body is not a malfunctioning machine. It is a brilliant, self-healing organism, and symptoms are sacred signals.

You were trained to distrust your body because a woman who trusts herself is hard to control.

A Brief History of Disempowerment

To understand how we got here, we have to go back. Long before pharmaceutical companies, healing was holistic. Rooted in Earth. Passed down through lineages. Women were the keepers of that knowledge, midwives, herbalists, energy workers, wise women.

And they were powerful.

Too powerful.

During the rise of patriarchy and industrialisation, female healers were branded as witches, heretics, and criminals. The burning times weren't just about fear of the occult, they were about eliminating natural, embodied knowledge. They were about replacing community led wellness with centralised control.

Enter: The Industrial Medical Complex.

By the early 1900s, powerhouses like the Rockefellers and Carnegies invested heavily in medical schools, funding education that favoured chemical based, patentable "medicine" and shunned anything they couldn't sell.

They rewrote the curriculum. They discredited herbalism, homeopathy, nutrition, and anything rooted in the Earth.

The Flexner Report of 1910 cemented the transformation of medicine from healing to business. And modern medicine, cold, clinical, detached, was born.

This system wasn't created to empower individuals. It was built to produce loyal, medicated consumers.

Symptoms as Currency

Let's talk about the economy of sickness.

The medical model is not designed to make you well. It is designed to keep you dependent.

Here's how the cycle works:

1. You feel unwell.
2. You're told it's normal, genetic, or chronic.
3. You're prescribed medication.
4. That medication causes side effects.
5. You're given more medication.
6. You're now on a cocktail of drugs that manage symptoms but cure nothing.
7. You're still sick. You're still tired. But now you're also disempowered, confused, and trapped.

Every repeat prescription is income. Every "routine" test, every follow-up, every re-prescription, it's all part of a billion-pound cycle.

Meanwhile, addressing the root cause, diet, sleep, trauma, nervous system regulation, toxic load, rarely gets a mention.

Why?

Because healing doesn't generate longterm revenue.
But management? Management is a goldmine.

And the most tragic part?
We were raised to think this was help.

The Obedience Conditioning

Most of us didn't enter adulthood sovereign.
We entered as well trained, obedient good girls.

From a young age, we learned how to trade truth for approval.
We weren't taught to listen, we were taught to obey.
We were praised for politeness, not curiosity.
We were told to follow rules, not question systems.

This was never more evident than in how we were taught to approach our bodies.

Instead of being taught to track our cycles, we were offered hormonal birth control as the default solution for "problem periods."
Instead of exploring the root of fatigue, mood swings, bloating, or acne, we were given synthetic Band-Aids and told to be grateful.
Instead of learning how nutrition, trauma, and the nervous system affect every part of our health, we were told to "lose weight" and "calm down."

The system doesn't want you aware. It wants you compliant.
And it uses shame as a control mechanism.

Shame as a Silencer

Here's the formula:

Make women ashamed of their bodies, and they'll never trust themselves enough to rise.

So they shamed:

Our bleeding.
Our hormones.
Our hunger.
Our tears.
Our sex drive.
Our intuition.
Our desire for rest.
Our desire for more.

They called us hormonal, hysterical, dramatic, irrational, too much.

They pathologised the exact things that make us powerful. And when our bodies spoke louder through symptoms, they offered silence in the form of medication.

We became afraid of our own biology. Afraid to ask questions.

Afraid to push back. Afraid to admit we still didn't feel right after being told we should be "fine." This shame doesn't belong to you. It was never yours. It was a tool of suppression.

And now? You get to release it.

The Gaslighting of the Feminine Body

Let's talk about the deep, unspoken epidemic in modern medicine: gaslighting.

Women are routinely dismissed, misdiagnosed, or ignored in clinical settings.

We're told our pain is exaggerated.
That our exhaustion is mental, not physical.
That our autoimmune flares are "probably just stress."
That our children's symptoms are imagined or overblown.
That our gut issues are all in our head.
That our hormonal chaos is just "part of being a woman."

This isn't an accident. This is a system designed around a male body template, in testing, treatment, and education.

Women are biologically different. We metabolise drugs differently. We experience illness differently. But that complexity? It's seen as inconvenient.

So instead of learning our rhythms, medicine tries to flatten them. Instead of working with our cycles, they medicate us into chemical suppression. Instead of exploring the energetic body, they fragment us into symptoms. Instead of seeing our emotions as signals, they brand them as disorders.
And when we dare to speak up? We're labelled as difficult, hysterical, hormonal, or noncompliant.

The Nervous System and Medical Trauma

Now, let's talk about the nervous system response to being gaslit and ignored.

When you repeatedly seek help and are dismissed, your body remembers. Your nervous system begins to associate medical care with threat not safety. This is medical trauma and it's real.

You may feel:

Dread when making appointments.
Panic before tests.
Numbness during conversations with healthcare providers.
Disbelief in your own symptoms.
Shame for "not speaking up enough."

It's not that you're weak, it's that your nervous system is trying to protect you from more harm. But healing begins when you start listening again.

When you regulate. When you breathe. When you validate your own experience. When you say: "My body is not lying. My intuition is not irrational. My symptoms are sacred."
You don't have to trust the system to trust yourself. And that's where true healing begins.

Pharmaceutical Influence & The Business of Sickness

Let's get brutally honest. The pharmaceutical industry isn't a healing system, it's a profit engine.

It doesn't thrive when you get well.
It thrives when you stay just unwell enough to require ongoing management.
It thrives when you need symptom relief, not root cause resolution.
It thrives when you come back every month for the refill, the test, the tweak.

And it doesn't want you empowered. It wants you dependent.

Dependent on the antidepressants, even though no one ever taught you to understand or support nervous system. Dependent on the pill, even though no one ever taught you to understand your cycle. Dependent on the prescriptions, even though no one asked what you eat, how you sleep, or how you feel in your body.

We've been told to praise the very system that keeps us sick. To be "good patients" even when we're getting worse. To be grateful we have options, even if they keep us numb, inflamed, bloated, exhausted, and silent.

And we're gaslit into believing anything outside this system is dangerous, unproven, or naive.

But here's what they don't want you to know:

You are allowed to ask questions. You are allowed to seek alternatives. You are allowed to walk away from what no longer serves your health.

Because this isn't healing. This is consumerism dressed up in a lab coat.

The Myth of "Evidence-Based" Medicine

One of the most effective spells cast by modern medicine is this phrase: "There's no evidence to support that." You'll hear it whenever you mention herbs, energy work, homeopathy, food as medicine, or detoxing your environment.

But let's talk about what "evidence-based" really means.

It means someone paid to fund the research. The research was published in a peer-reviewed journal. It followed a format acceptable to mainstream science (usually short-term, reductionist, and designed to isolate variables). And ideally, the treatment being studied can be commercialised.

So if no one's funding large studies on mugwort or yarrow or seed cycling or EFT tapping or breathwork or trauma healing, does that mean they're not valid?

Of course not.

It means there's no profit in proving them. It means ancient wisdom doesn't play well in capitalist systems. You are allowed to value evidence that comes from experience, not just spreadsheets.

You are allowed to trust centuries of herbal knowledge, ancestral rituals, and intuitive healing, even if no man in a lab coat has signed off on it.

That's not reckless. That's reclamation.

Fear Marketing and Wellness Dependency

Now let's talk about another layer of control: fear-based wellness.

Once women start waking up to the brokenness of conventional medicine, they often fall headfirst into a different trap, the wellness industry.
Where pharmaceuticals sell dependency on prescriptions, the wellness industry can sell dependency on products.

Suddenly, you're told you need:

27 supplements a day.
An expensive detox protocol.
A new guru.
A fancy tool.
A specific spiritual practice.
A £300 a month subscription.
A brand-new nervous system regulation method every week.

And if you don't do it all, you're not "serious" about your healing. If you don't have the budget, you're to blame for not getting better. If your symptoms persist, it must be your mindset.

See how the shame cycle creeps back in?

You went from obedient patient to overwhelmed wellness consumer. Same pattern. Different packaging.

But true sovereignty isn't found in products. It's found in presence.

You don't need everything.
You need alignment.
You need education.
You need nervous system safety.
You need community.
You need truth.

And you already hold more wisdom than any brand can sell you.

Ancestral Disconnection: The Broken Lineage

Before we ever questioned the system, our grandmothers lived it.

Many of them held the threads of natural wisdom, sometimes consciously, sometimes in fragments.

The hot compress on the belly for period pain.
The nettle tea in spring for vitality.
The way they knew when someone was "off" without words.
The stories they told that no one wrote down.
The remedies they offered without diagnosis.

But many of them were never allowed to own that wisdom.

They were told to hush.
To modernise.
To sterilise their instincts.
To defer to their husbands.
To stop "being silly."
To abandon the old ways.

Some of them survived trauma we can barely imagine. War. Poverty. Miscarriage. Stillbirth. Abuse. Loss. And they were offered medication, religion, and obedience in place of actual healing.

They handed us what they could, but so many of the threads were cut. And now? You are the weaver.

You are the one holding the needle and thread, standing at the threshold between what was and what can be.

The system told them to forget. But you? You are here to remember. You Were Born for This Work You feel it in your bones, don't you?

That what you're doing now isn't just for you. It's for the daughters who come next. It's for the ancestors who weren't allowed to speak.

Your healing is a return, not a reinvention.

When you light that candle and blend that tea, you're not just trying to feel better. You're reclaiming lost rites. When you say no to that prescription that never felt right, you're breaking the silence. When you choose to rest, cry, scream, or research, you are repairing the lineage.

You may be the first woman in your line to say:

"That's not good enough."
"There has to be another way."
"I trust my body."
"I deserve real healing."
"No more silence. No more shame."
"The cycle ends here."

That's not a trend.
That's a soul contract.
You are the sacred disruptor.
The healer your bloodline has been waiting for.

Building Your Own Healing System

So how do you begin? How do you actually opt out of a system designed to keep you in?

You start by making micro choices that align with your sovereignty.

You start small, but you start powerfully.

1. Detox your home, not just your body.

Every product you swap is a rebellion.
Choose low toxin alternatives when you can.
Start with the things you use daily, cleaners, laundry, deodorant, toothpaste.
Let your home become a healing space.

2. Get curious, not compliant.

Ask questions. Always.
Why this test? Why this medication? What are the side effects?
What are the other options?
If they roll their eyes, you're in the right place.

3. Track your cycle.

Learn your rhythm. Know your seasons. Understand how your body shifts across the month.
It is your compass, and it holds more diagnostic power than most blood tests.

4. Support your nervous system daily.

Regulation isn't a luxury, it's foundational.
Prioritise breathwork, somatics, slow movement, music, nature, connection.
You don't have to meditate for an hour a day. You just have to take a moment to connect to the safety of your body.

5. Reconnect with the Earth.

Barefoot in the grass.
Mugwort in the bath.
Lavender on your pillow.
Let the Earth be your pharmacy.
She always was.

6. Know your healing is layered.

You are physical, emotional, energetic, ancestral, and spiritual.
No system that ignores your multidimensionality can ever fully heal you.

You're Not Alone.

You are not doing this work in isolation. Right now, all over the world, women are waking up. Ditching their pills. Reading ingredient labels. Learning how to make their own tinctures.

Questioning their birth plans. Reclaiming their rage. Tending their wombs. Teaching their children what they were never taught.

We are not scattered.
We are a forest.
Connected underground.
Unseen by those who live in the towers.
But mighty.
Unstoppable.
And growing.

The sacred rebellion is rising.
And you, dear one, are part of the storm.

What Sovereignty Looks Like in Action

Let's strip away the fluff. Sovereignty is not a vibe, it's a daily decision.

It's how you breathe before saying yes.
It's how you speak up when your body says no.
It's how you listen to the whispers before they become screams.

Sovereignty doesn't mean you never use medication.
It doesn't mean you live in a yurt off-grid and forage your food.

It means you choose, from an empowered place, not fear, not programming, not compliance.

It means:

You take the antibiotics if you decide they're the right tool, not because you were pressured.
You skip the vaccine, or you don't, but you make the decision based on your body, your research, your truth.
You work with a doctor who respects your voice, or you fire the one who doesn't.

It's not black or white.
It's not "alternative" vs. "conventional."
It's sovereign vs. submissive.

And your body knows the difference.

A Ritual for Reclamation

This ritual is simple, but potent. You can do it today, tonight, next moon, whenever it feels needed.

Ritual: The Sovereignty Anointing

You'll need:

- A candle
- A journal
- A natural oil or herbal salve (bonus points if you made it yourself or know the plant)

1. Light your candle.
2. Anoint your wrists, belly, and heart with your oil or salve.
3. Close your eyes. Breathe deep into your body.
4. Whisper or speak aloud:

"I no longer surrender my health to systems that profit from my silence.
I reclaim my body.
I reclaim my intuition.
I reclaim my medicine.
I walk in truth, not obedience.
I choose sovereignty, daily, gently, radically."

Let the oil absorb. Let the words land. Let the old patterns fall away.

You are not asking for permission anymore.
You are crowning yourself.

Sacred Journal Prompts

These are designed to go deep. Let them pull truth from your marrow.

Where in my life am I still outsourcing my authority?
What does "informed choice" really mean to me?
How have I silenced myself to be a "good patient" or a "good girl"?
What would it look like to fully rebuild trust with my body?
Where do I need to forgive myself for choices I made before I knew better?
What does sovereignty feel like in my body, not just my mind?
Who or what do I need to release to step fully into empowered healing?

Write. Cry. Rage. Dance. Let your nervous system metabolise the truth. This is not about having the right answers. It's about remembering that you get to ask the questions.

The Spell is Broken. You Are the Medicine.

This chapter began with a reckoning.
It ends with a rebirth.
You are no longer just someone trying to "get better."
You are a living revolution.

When you question the system, you challenge centuries of control.
When you regulate your nervous system, you disrupt cycles of trauma.
When you honour your symptoms, you reclaim sacred communication.
When you trust your body, you dismantle generational gaslighting.

And when you choose sovereignty, you light a fire in others to do the same.

Let them watch you glow. Let them ask how you did it.
Let them feel the quiet quake of a woman who knows herself.

Because now you're not looking for healing. You are walking it.

Chapter 3

The Poison in the Products

Your home is either your first healing sanctuary, or your slowest source of suffering. There's something insidious about this part of the awakening.

You can prepare yourself to question the medical system.
You can brace for the pushback when you ditch prescriptions or call out gaslighting.

But no one tells you how hard it hits when you realise the things you trusted the most, your shampoo, your washing powder, your baby's bubble bath, are harming you quietly, daily, and legally.

The betrayal cuts deep. Because these are the things you brought into your home with good intentions.
The "sensitive skin" brands. The baby safe soaps. The "dermatologist recommended" lotions.

The products that came with smiling mothers on the packaging and soft pastel branding.

And yet, inside those bottles?
Carcinogens.
Endocrine disruptors.
Neurotoxins.
All approved. All normalised. All marketed with love.

Welcome to the part of the spell they hope you never break:
The toxin trap inside your home.

The Invisible Load

Before you knew, you used what everyone else did.

You filled your home with fabric softener and bleach.
You wiped down the high chair with disinfectant wipes.
You sprayed air freshener before guests arrived.
You put baby lotion on fresh skin, thinking it was gentle.
You trusted the words on the label. "Pure." "Clean." "Safe."

You didn't know these terms meant nothing.
You didn't know those scents were synthetic and unregulated.
You didn't know the damage was cumulative.
You didn't know it would build up in your womb, your liver, your breast milk, your children.

And now? Now you do.
And when you know, you cannot unknow.

You're Not Crazy: You're Contaminated

Let's be blunt: most of us have never known what it feels like to live in a body not under chemical assault.

From the womb, we are absorbing:

Phthalates from plastic.
Parabens from skincare.
Formaldehyde from baby wipes.
Synthetic fragrance from cleaning sprays.
Aluminium from deodorant.
Fluoride from toothpaste.
PFAS from cookware.
Glyphosate from food.
VOCs from paint, carpets, furniture.

And the result?

Fatigue.
Brain fog.
Hormonal imbalance.
Reproductive issues.

Chronic inflammation.
Autoimmune flares.
Allergies.
Anxiety.
Even infertility.

And we're told it's just modern life.
Or that we're "just sensitive."
Or that it's genetic.

No. It's exposure. It's accumulation. It's systemic chemical warfare marketed as convenience.

A Culture Built on Toxins

Let's zoom out. After WWII, industries had a massive surplus of chemicals. And so they found a new market: the household.

Leftover nerve gas compounds were repurposed into pesticides.
Industrial solvents became air fresheners.
Rocket fuel derivatives were added to shampoo.
Petrochemicals entered beauty products en masse.

The FDA, the EPA, the UK's regulatory equivalents? They allowed it. Still do. Because the system prioritises profit over purity.

Most ingredients on shelves today have never been tested for long-term safety in humans, especially in combination.
And it's not a conspiracy. It's policy.

You Are Not Overreacting. You Are Waking Up.

So no, you're not crazy for wanting to throw everything in your bathroom into the bin.

You're not paranoid for not trusting mainstream brands.
You're not dramatic for reading every label.
You're not over the top for refusing to put that bubble bath on your child.
You're not being "extra" for throwing out the Febreze.

You are taking your power back.
You are reclaiming your home as a healing space.
You are no longer letting the system poison you quietly.

And that? That is the deepest kind of rebellion.

Endocrine Disruptors: The Silent Saboteurs of the Feminine Body

Let's talk hormones. Because if you have a womb, cycles, breasts, or ever plan to carry life, you need to know what's in your environment.

Endocrine disruptors are chemicals that interfere with your body's natural hormonal communication.
They mimic, block, or alter how hormones are produced, released, or received in the body. And they are everywhere.

They show up in:

Plastic water bottles.
Food packaging.
Candles and air fresheners.
Deodorants and sunscreens.
Sanitary products.
Makeup.
Baby wipes.
Cleaning sprays.

And what do they do?

They destabilise your cycle.
They cause early puberty.
They worsen PMDD, endometriosis, and PCOS.
They mess with your fertility.
They increase your risk of breast, ovarian, and thyroid cancers.
They confuse your body's ability to regulate fat, insulin, sleep, and sex hormones.
They are a major reason we're seeing more hormonal disorders, reproductive issues, and unexplained fatigue than ever before.

But instead of addressing that root, we're offered more synthetic solutions:

The pill for heavy bleeding.
Antidepressants for PMS.
IVF for infertility.
HRT for early menopause.

And the cycle continues.
We are managing what we are being poisoned into experiencing.

Greenwashing & the "Clean" Lie

You finally start waking up. You ditch your big-name products. You reach for something "natural." And you grab the bottle that says:

"Organic"
"Hypoallergenic"
"Eco-Friendly"
"For sensitive skin"
"Plant-based"
"Pure"
"Dermatologist-approved"
"Fragrance-free"

But here's the truth: none of these labels are regulated.

A brand can add one drop of aloe vera to a formula full of toxins and call it "natural."
They can add synthetic fragrance and still slap on "clean."
They can use marketing words to lull you into safety, because they know that's what you want to see.

This is called greenwashing, and it's designed to manipulate your awakening. If you don't flip that bottle over and read the ingredients, you're relying on marketing, not truth.

Room by Room: Where Toxins Hide in Plain Sight

Let's take a sacred walk through your home. Not with fear, but with clarity.

BATHROOM

Shampoo & Conditioner: SLS, parabens, artificial fragrance
Toothpaste: Fluoride, PEGs, synthetic sweeteners
Deodorant: Aluminium, propylene glycol, triclosan
Pads & Tampons: Bleached cotton, dioxins, plastic
Makeup: Talc, PFAS, parabens, phthalates

KITCHEN

Tupperware: BPA/BPS leaching into food
Cookware: Non-stick pans (Teflon = PFAS)

Cleaning sprays: Ammonia, chlorine, formaldehyde
Dish soap: SLS, synthetic dyes, fragrance
Food storage: Plastic wrap, lined cans

LAUNDRY ROOM

Detergent: Optical brighteners, fragrance, 1,4 dioxane
Fabric softener: Quats, synthetic scent, petroleum-based chemicals
Dryer sheets: Endocrine disruptors disguised as "fresh scent"

LIVING ROOM & BEDROOM

Candles & wax melts: Paraffin wax, artificial scent, benzene
Air fresheners: Phthalates, formaldehyde, mystery fragrance
Furniture: Flame retardants, off gassing chemicals
Mattresses & bedding: VOCs, formaldehyde, synthetic fibres

Now breathe. This isn't about panic. This is about power.
You can't change what you don't see. But now? You see.

Your Home is a Temple, Not a Toxic Waste Site

There is nothing ordinary about your home. It is not just a roof. Not just four walls. It is an energetic container. A living altar. A sacred space where healing either flourishes or fails to.

When your environment is loaded with low vibrational, synthetic, and endocrine disruptive products, your nervous system knows. Even if your conscious mind is used to it. Even if the smell of that fabric softener feels nostalgic.

Your body still responds.
Your cells still recoil.
Your nervous system still flinches.

Toxic products lower the frequency of your space and by extension, your body.

So when you clear them out, you're not just detoxing your air, your skin, your bloodstream...
You're clearing stagnation.
You're removing spells of submission.
You're reclaiming spiritual sovereignty from the inside out.

Detox as a Spiritual Practice

Detox isn't just about being healthy. It's about choosing consciousness over convenience. It's about remembering that your body is a holy vessel, not a corporate dumping ground.

When you pour bleach into your toilet bowl, you're not just cleaning, you're saturating your home in harsh chemicals that alter your air, your skin, your gut, your hormones.

When you light a synthetic candle, you're not just creating ambiance, you're filling your sacred space with petrochemicals.

And when you choose not to do those things anymore? When you reach for herbs, essential oils, salt, vinegar, sunshine, plants, you are rejoining the ancient rhythm. You are making your home a healing ecosystem again. You are choosing to remember.

Every swap is a ceremony.
Every decluttering is an unbinding.
Every natural cleaner is an invocation of clarity.
Every time you choose presence over programming, you are activating your sacred rebellion.

Start Where You Are, Not Where You Think You Should Be

This can feel overwhelming at first. You look at your shelves and suddenly see everything differently. The mascara. The hand soap. The cupboard of "cleaning" sprays. The lotions. The wipes. The makeup. It can feel like everything needs to go. And maybe, eventually, it will.

But please hear this:

You do not need to fix it all overnight.
You do not need to spend hundreds on new products today.

You are not behind. You are not failing.

You are beginning.

Start with what you use the most.
Start with what touches your skin daily.
Start with your bed, your body, your breath.
Start with the products that feel most intuitively wrong.

Let your swaps be sacred, not stressful. Let your rhythm of change be intuitive, not panicked. This is not about becoming another kind of consumer, it's about becoming conscious.

The Energetic Cost of Toxicity

Everything has a frequency. And many of the products we've used for years carry the energetic frequency of:

Suppression.
Control.
Numbness.
Compliance.
Disconnection.

You can feel it when you walk into someone's home. You can smell the artificial scent before you see the synthetic décor. You can sense when a space is heavy, even if it's spotless.

Now imagine walking into a space that smells of cedarwood, lavender, lemon balm. Where there are no aerosol sprays but instead windows cracked open for fresh air. Where there are plants cleansing the air, salt lamps softening the light, and handmade oils blessing the skin.

That is not just a toxin free space.
That is a frequency raising temple.
That is a homecoming.

And you don't need a big house, money, or Pinterest perfection to create it. You just need to start saying no more poison, and yes to presence.

Practical Detox Swaps (and Why They Matter Energetically)

Let's get real: this isn't about chasing perfection.
It's about making conscious, intentional swaps that radically shift the energy of your home and the health of your body.

Here are some foundational swaps that pack a powerful punch, physically and spiritually:

1. Fabric Softener → White Vinegar + Essential Oils

Why: Fabric softeners contain endocrine disruptors, synthetic fragrance, and petroleum-based compounds.

Swap energy: From synthetic masking to natural purification. Vinegar clears stagnant energy. Lavender, lemon, or eucalyptus oils raise vibration while softening fabric.

2. Scented Candles → Beeswax or Soy Candles / Oil Diffusers

Why: Most candles release benzene and toluene, neurotoxic compounds.

Swap energy: Beeswax purifies air and has ancient ceremonial roots. Diffusing essential oils sets intentional tone, calming, grounding, awakening.

3. Bleach & Harsh Cleaners → White Vinegar, Castile Soap, Bicarb + Essential Oils

Why: Chemical cleaners harm lungs, skin, hormones, and kill good bacteria.

Swap energy: You shift from sterile control to harmonious cleansing. Think rosemary for protection, citrus for clarity, peppermint for mental focus.

4. Conventional Skincare → Herbal Balms, Infused Oils, Clean Formulations

Why: Lotions are often full of parabens, alcohols, and synthetic stabilisers.

Swap energy: Skin is sacred, choose formulations that nourish the barrier and honour the ritual. Your skincare becomes a moment of connection, not a chemical assault.

5. Plastic Water Bottles → Glass or Stainless Steel

Why: Plastics leach hormone disruptors into your water, especially when warm.

Swap energy: Drinking from glass is energetically clean, structurally sound, and symbolically transparent. Your hydration becomes intentional.

These swaps aren't just about ingredients. They're about identity. You're no longer someone who just consumes, you're someone who creates environments of wellness.

Each swap is a boundary. A statement. A spell breaking.

Homemaking as Ancestral Healing

You weren't taught this part in school. You weren't taught that making your own cleaning spray could connect you to your grandmother's forgotten wisdom. That crafting salves and tinctures is holy work. That boiling herbs on the stove for air cleansing is older than any aerosol. That scrubbing your floor with rosemary and salt is spellwork. That folding sheets scented with lavender oil is an act of love your ancestors feel.

We live in a culture that mocks the sacredness of homemaking, but for many women, this is where the reclamation begins. It is not about being domestic. It is about remembering that every part of your environment is alive with meaning.

Your home is not a side note to your healing. It's the first chapter.

A Ritual for Clearing, Cleansing, and Reclaiming

You'll need:

- A bowl of hot water
- A handful of rosemary or lavender
- A few drops of essential oil
- A cloth or broom

- Salt (any kind)

1. Prepare your space. Open windows. Light a candle. Ground.

2. Add herbs and oils to the bowl. Let it steep. This is your sacred cleansing water.

3. Dip your cloth or broom into the mixture. As you wipe or sweep each room, say aloud:

*"I clear what no longer belongs.
I cleanse what has been unseen.
I welcome in the sacred.
This space remembers me, and I remember it."*

4. Sprinkle a pinch of salt at each doorway. Protection. Boundary. Blessing.

5. When you're done, pour the water outside with gratitude. Let the Earth transmute what was released.

Sacred Journal Prompts

What products in my home carry energy that no longer feels aligned?
Where am I still holding onto things "just in case" or from guilt?
What does a healing home feel, smell, and look like to me?

What old beliefs about cleaning, beauty, or home am I ready to release?
What ancestral wisdom wants to return through my homemaking?

What Clean Living Really Means (And What It Doesn't)

Let's be honest: the words clean living have been co-opted.

They've been filtered through Instagram aesthetics and wellness trends that make it look like you need a £10,000 kitchen, a minimalist white house, and a cabinet full of adaptogens to qualify.
Let's redefine it. Clean living isn't about perfection. It's about presence.

It means:

You are conscious of what enters your space.
You read labels, not because you're paranoid, but because you're powerful.
You make swaps as you're able, not out of fear, but from sovereignty.
You prioritise frequency over formula.
You know that what you allow into your home is either nourishing your nervous system, or numbing your intuition.

Clean living isn't about being toxin free. That's nearly impossible in this world.

It's about reducing your load so your body has a chance to return to wisdom.

It's about choosing to clear the path.
So your hormones can stabilise.
Your sleep can deepen.
Your children can breathe easier.
Your home can become a temple.
Your truth can get louder.

Living Low-Toxin Without Fear

Let's say this now, for your nervous system:

You do not need to live in fear of every item in your house.
You do not need to throw everything away tomorrow.
You do not need to panic every time someone brings over a store bought hand soap.
Fear is not the frequency we are building your rebellion in.

We are building it in:

Truth.
Discernment.
Choice.
Compassion.
Gradual, sustainable change.

Your body doesn't need perfection. It needs a break.

And every product you choose to replace, every chemical you remove, every synthetic scent you no longer welcome, is a break. A break in the chain. A crack in the system. A clearing of your field.

You don't need to be pure. You just need to be present.

Final Integration: Your Body, Your Home, Your Medicine

You are the medicine. Your hands, your choices, your breath, your presence, are what heals.

When you make a balm, you are not just making skincare. You are alchemising safety.
When you mop the floor with salt and lemon oil, you are not just cleaning, you are clearing trauma.

When you open the window instead of spraying air freshener, you are not just airing out the room, you are calling your soul back in.
This is what they never taught us.
That healing lives in the mundane.
That detoxing our homes is spiritual reclamation.
That homemaking is resistance.
That every low toxin choice is a spell of sovereignty.

You're not doing this alone.
You're part of a quiet revolution.
One bottle. One breath. One boundary at a time.

And now?

Your home remembers.
Your body responds.
And the rebellion deepens.

Ritual: Anchoring Clean Power

You'll need:

- A small bowl of water
- A sprig of fresh herb (or a pinch of dried rosemary, basil, lavender, bay, anything sacred to you)
- Your breath

Stir the herb into the water.
Hold it in your hands.
Say:

"May I cleanse what dims my truth.
May I clear what clouds my knowing.
May I create a space that remembers what I came here to become."

Flick the water at your doorstep, in your bathroom, on your altar, or pour it into your plants.

This is your threshold.
This is your line in the sand.
No more poison.
No more pretending.
You choose clarity now.

Resources to Support a Clean Lifestyle

Recommended Books

This Is Your Brain on Birth Control – Dr. Sarah E. Hill.
Explores how hormonal birth control affects mood, cognition, and health.

Estrogeneration – **Dr. Anthony G. Jay.** Unpacks the epidemic of hormone-disrupting chemicals in our daily lives and how they impact fertility, mood, and metabolism.

The Non-Tinfoil Guide to EMFs – **Nicolas Pineault.** Simple, science-backed exploration of electromagnetic pollution and its biological impact.

Toxic Beauty – **Samuel S. Epstein & Randall Fitzgerald.** A deep dive into harmful ingredients in cosmetics and personal care products.

Slow Death by Rubber Duck – **Rick Smith & Bruce Lourie.** Two environmentalists test how everyday exposure to toxins shows up in their bodies. Eye-opening and relatable.

The Autoimmune Solution – **Dr. Amy Myers.** Links environmental toxins to the rise in autoimmune conditions and offers a natural healing path.

Documentaries & Films

Stink! **(Netflix / Amazon).** Tracks a father's investigation into fragrance ingredients after his daughter's pyjamas arrive smelling weird. Exposes the cosmetics loophole.

The Human Experiment. Explores the silent rise of hormone-related illness due to chemical exposure.

Dark Waters. Based on a true story, exposes DuPont's coverup of toxic PFAS chemicals (Teflon).

Unacceptable Levels. A personal and powerful look at the thousands of chemicals in our environment and their links to disease.

Websites & Tools

EWG.org (Environmental Working Group)

- Skin Deep Database (check your cosmetics).
- Tap Water Database.
- Guide to Clean Cleaning Products.
- Food Scores.

Think Dirty App

Scan your products to check for harmful ingredients. Great for skincare and household swaps.

Made Safe Certified

Directory of verified non-toxic products.

Dr. Mark Hyman's Podcast – "The Doctor's Farmacy"

Especially episodes on toxins, detox, and functional medicine insights.

Chapter 4

The Body Remembers

Your symptoms are not a malfunction, they're a message.
You've been taught your whole life that your body is a problem to solve.

From the moment your period arrived, you were handed painkillers. When your skin broke out, you were told to scrub harder and medicate faster. When you felt anxious, you were told to "calm down." When you gained weight, you were told to shrink. When you expressed pain, you were told it was normal.

And when the symptoms piled up? When you couldn't get out of bed? When your cycle went rogue, your gut turned against you, your skin scared, your brain fogged?

You were told your body was failing you. But what if she wasn't failing? What if she was speaking? What if every pain, every rash, every ache, every imbalance, was a breadcrumb leading you back to yourself?

Not Broken Just Misread

You are not broken. You are misinterpreted. Not just by others, but by yourself, because that's what you were trained to do.

We live in a world that encourages disembodiment. We're taught to live from the neck up, logic, language, lists. But your body? She speaks in sensations, instincts, pulses, and symptoms.

When you get a headache, she's not attacking you. She's asking you to listen.
When your period arrives early and painful, she's not punishing you. She's processing something.
When your digestion slows, ares, bloats, she's not being difficult. She's alerting you to overload.

Your body isn't resisting healing. She's revealing what still needs to be held.

Symptoms as Sacred Signals

Let's ip the script:

Fatigue isn't laziness. It's a full body no to pushing beyond your limits.
Bloating isn't bad digestion, it's unprocessed emotion, poor boundaries, or toxic overload.

Anxiety isn't dysfunction, it's your nervous system trying to keep you safe.
Hormonal acne isn't random, it's your internal ecosystem begging for rebalance.
Brain fog isn't just stress, it's disconnection, inflammation, and information overwhelm.

Your body doesn't use words. She uses symptoms. And she will escalate the volume until you pay attention.

This isn't punishment. This is communication.

You Weren't Taught to Speak the Language

When was the last time someone said, "Let's get curious about what your body is trying to say?"

Probably never.

Because that's not how this system works. You were taught to suppress, silence, override, distract. You were taught to fear pain, numb emotion, and keep functioning.

But when you ignore your body's signals, you disconnect from your inner guidance system. You lose the ability to feel truth in your gut. You stop trusting your cravings. You override your intuitive no. You confuse disassociation for peace. You become more afraid of symptoms than of staying misaligned.

But here's the good news:

It's not too late to learn the language of your body. She's still speaking. She never gave up on you.

The Energetic Roots of Illness

The body doesn't lie.
She doesn't sugar coat.
She doesn't rationalise or gaslight.
She doesn't care about your calendar, your deadlines, or your plans.

She cares about truth. And when truth is buried, dismissed, or repressed, it doesn't disappear. It finds a home. In your joints. Your womb. Your gut. Your jaw. Your skin.
Every place your body holds tight is a place your story hasn't been allowed to breathe.

Western medicine might call it "inflammation" or "stress." But in sacred medicine, we call it unmetabolised emotion. Frozen energy. Suppressed memory. Cellular story.
We are taught to treat pain like it's the enemy. But what if pain is actually your body's deepest form of honesty?

Trauma Doesn't Just Live in the Mind

Trauma isn't just what happens to you, it's what happens inside you as a result. And where does that energy go when it has nowhere to land?

Into the nervous system. Into the fascia. Into the womb.

Let's break that down.

1. The Nervous System: Your Internal Surveillance System

When you experienced trauma, whether medical, emotional, physical, or spiritual, your body responded. Your nervous system went into overdrive.

Fight. Flight. Freeze. Fawn.

And if you didn't have the tools, time, or safety to complete the cycle? That energy stayed trapped. You stayed in a low grade survival loop.

You got good at functioning, but never feeling safe.
And chronic dysregulation leads to symptoms:

Anxiety

Digestive issues
Sleep disturbances
Immune imbalances
Hormonal chaos

You're not just anxious. Your body may still be carrying signals from times when it wasn't safe to feel what was true in that moment.

2. Fascia: The Body's Emotional Memory Bank

Fascia is the connective tissue that wraps around every muscle, bone, and organ. It's often called the "second nervous system" because it holds emotional memory.

Have you ever cried during a deep stretch?
Felt waves of emotion during bodywork?
Experienced grief come up during yoga?

That's fascia releasing stored trauma.
This is why body-based healing isn't optional, it's essential.

3. The Womb: Your Seat of Creation and Storage

The womb is where you create, hold, release, and store. It is one of the most intuitive parts of the female body. And it is also one of the most colonised.

Painful periods, broids, endometriosis, infertility, these are not random.

They are often:

A response to unexpressed grief.
A build-up of ancestral trauma.
A consequence of chronic suppression.
A reaction to environmental toxins.
A plea for reconnection.

Your womb remembers every time you didn't feel safe to speak.
Every boundary you couldn't hold.
Every time you said yes when your body said no.

But she also remembers joy. Pleasure. Creativity. Power.

You are not broken, you are holding too much. And that can change.

The Myth of Random Illness

One of the most dangerous narratives in modern medicine is this:

"We don't know what causes it. It's probably genetic. You'll have it for life."

The Sacred Rebellion

This statement is not truth. It's pause in curiosity. It can leave us feeling powerless and disconnected from our own healing process and dependent on management rather than supported in deeper understanding.

Yes some conditions do have genetic components, but your genes are not a fixed fate.

Epigenetics is showing us that our experiences, including stress, trauma, environment, nourishment, nervous system patterns, even relationships and belonging can influence how genes are expressed.

Illness doesn't appear in a vacuum, it often carries context, physical, emotional, generational. Sometimes it's the body's way of asking us to listen more deeply not because we've failed, but because it is wise.

It is your body's last resort when all other messages have been ignored. It is an intelligent, protective response to a world that was never designed for your full aliveness.

Your illness is not your identity. It's your body's language of truth.

Decoding Common Symptoms Holistically

Let's explore how symptoms carry multiple layers of meaning, physical, emotional, energetic, and spiritual.

Fatigue

Physical: Adrenal fatigue, blood sugar dysregulation, toxic overload.
Emotional: Burnout from overgiving, people-pleasing, emotional suppression.
Energetic: Lack of boundaries, energy leaks, carrying others' pain
Message: You are carrying too much that was never yours. Rest is not weakness, it is wisdom.

Digestive Issues (bloating, IBS, constipation, reflux)

Physical: Imbalanced microbiome, food intolerances, poor vagal tone.
Emotional: Unprocessed stress, "gut feelings" ignored, self-rejection.
Energetic: Lack of safety, blocked solar plexus, boundary breaches.
Message: What are you not digesting emotionally? What truth are you struggling to process?

Acne / Skin Issues

Physical: Detox pathways overwhelmed, hormonal imbalance, inflammatory food triggers.
Emotional: Shame, visibility fears, inner criticism.
Energetic: Self-protection, fear of being seen, old identity shedding.
Message: What is trying to rise to the surface? What truth or identity wants to be witnessed?

Headaches / Migraines

Physical: Tension, blood sugar drops, dehydration, chemical sensitivity.
Emotional: Pressure to perform, perfectionism, overstimulation
Energetic: Crowded crown chakra, blocked intuition.
Message: What are you trying to "think" your way through instead of feeling? What pressure are you holding that isn't yours?

Painful Periods / Womb Conditions

Physical: Estrogen dominance, inflammation, stagnation.
Emotional: Suppressed creativity, womb grief, generational trauma.
Energetic: Disconnection from feminine power, misaligned creation.
Message: What creative force is trying to move through you?

What has your womb been asked to hold that was never hers to carry?

This is just the beginning. Your symptoms are unique. And your body is not asking for punishment, it's asking for partnership.

Creating a Sacred Conversation with Your Body

You don't need to be urgent in medical terminology. You need to become urgent in your body's language.

Start simple:

When a symptom arises, pause.
Ask: "What are you trying to tell me?"
Place your hand over the area.
Breathe into it.
Say: "I'm listening."
Journal what arises.
Even if it makes no sense yet, write it down.
Track patterns.

What ares up when you're stressed?
When you're in certain environments?
With certain people?

Treat every symptom like a letter from your inner self.

Read it with curiosity, not judgment.
Ask it what it needs, not how to silence it.
Respond with compassion, not control.

This is the foundation of embodied sovereignty.

From Suppression to Sovereignty

The old way told you to silence, numb, override.

Pop a pill.
Power through.
Push harder.
Be grateful it's not worse.
Don't make a fuss.

But the sacred rebellion whispers something different.
Listen. Soften. Slow down. Partner with the body.
Sovereignty doesn't mean never having symptoms.
It means choosing how you respond to them.

Instead of fear? You respond with curiosity.
Instead of control? You offer compassion.
Instead of panic? You ground into presence.

That's the moment sovereignty is born, not in the absence of pain, but in the choice to meet it consciously.

Healing Begins With Safety

Your body will not heal in a state of threat.
Even the most powerful herbs, protocols, and therapies won't land if your nervous system is locked in survival mode.

This is why safety must come first.
You do not need to feel safe all the time.
You simply need moments of safety.

Small anchors. Sacred pauses.
Nervous system signals that say, "We're okay right now."

Here are daily acts of safety that begin rewiring your body's trust:

Laying at on the floor, hand on heart, breathing deeply for 3 minutes.
Saying "thank you" to a part of your body, even the part that hurts.
Massaging your jaw or your womb while listening to calming music.
Creating a morning ritual that involves no screens, just self.
Drinking warm herbal tea with both hands, and simply... being.
Each act says: "I'm not here to fight you. I'm here to listen."
That's where healing starts.

Daily Embodiment is a Rebellion

We've been trained to live outside of our bodies.
We've been rewarded for numbing, ignoring, pushing past.

But the world doesn't need more women disconnected from their flesh. The world needs more women rooted.

Rooted in breath.
Rooted in cycle.
Rooted in rhythm.
Rooted in truth.

So how do you return?

By coming back into your body daily, not as a task, but as a devotion.

Let embodiment be:

Movement that feels good, not punishing.
Nourishment that honours your inner landscape.
Stillness that recalibrates your energy.
Sounds that awaken your cells.
Pleasure that reminds you you're alive.
This isn't about aesthetic wellness.
This is about liberation.

Your body is your rebellion. And every time you choose presence over programming, she celebrates.

A Ritual for Body Listening

You don't need a diagnosis to begin healing.
You need a relationship with your body.
And relationships begin with conversation.

This ritual invites you into sacred dialogue with your physical self.

Ritual: The Body Oracle

You'll need:

- A quiet space
- A journal
- A blanket
- Optional: a crystal or herbal oil (lavender, rose, or mugwort are beautiful choices)

1. Get comfortable. Lie down or sit, wrapped in your blanket. Let your body soften.
2. Close your eyes. Place your hands on the part of your body that speaks to you most. It might be where there's pain. It might be where you feel disconnected. It might just be your heart.

3. Breathe deeply. Ask: "What are you holding?" Don't try to x. Just listen.

4. When ready, ask: "What do you need from me?" Let images, memories, sensations, or words rise. Trust what you receive.

5. Journal it all. Every whisper. Every feeling. Every resistance.

6. When complete, thank your body. Say out loud:

"I choose to listen.
I choose to stay.
I choose to trust you again."

You are now in sacred partnership.

Sacred Journal Prompts

What symptoms have I been fighting that are really just messages I haven't translated yet?
Where do I override my body's truth out of habit, fear, or pressure?
What emotion is living in the part of my body that hurts the most?

The Sacred Rebellion

What would it feel like to be fully at home in my body again?
How can I begin treating my body as a living oracle, not a broken machine?

You Are the Oracle

The rebellion isn't about mastering every health protocol or becoming a wellness expert.
It's about remembering that the deepest, wisest guidance lives inside you.

Your body is your compass.
Your symptoms are your signals.
Your intuition is your language.
Your presence is your power.

This chapter isn't about xing the body, it's about coming home to her.

Because she was never the enemy. She was the map all along.

And now? You're reading it. You're learning her dialect.
And with every breath, every choice, every sacred pause…
You are rewriting the story.

Chapter 5

Rewilding the Feminine

You were not born to be tame. You were born to be untethered, undomesticated, and unapologetically alive.

There's a wildness inside you.

It shows up when your blood comes.
When you scream into your pillow instead of smiling through it.
When you dance in the kitchen barefoot with no one watching.
When you rage, cry, bleed, laugh, create, or collapse into the arms of the Earth.

It's the part of you that doesn't ask for permission.
The part that never cared about being polite.
The part that remembers herbs, ancestors, and full moon nights.
The part that howls when something isn't right, and knows exactly how to make it right again.

That wildness? She never left.

She was just buried under layers of obedience, shame, and productivity. This chapter is about bringing her back.

The Taming of the Feminine

You weren't born tame.

As a baby, you cried when you needed.
As a child, you spoke what you saw.
You were curious. Sensual. Loud. Emotional. Unfiltered.

And then?
You were taught to tone it down.

"Don't cry."
"Don't be silly."
"Be quiet."
"Be good."
"Cover up."
"Don't take up space."
"That's not ladylike."
"You're being dramatic."
"You're too sensitive."
"You're too loud."
"You're too much."

So you started shrinking. Not just your voice, but your instinct. You questioned your own emotions. You tried to be liked instead of being true. You moulded yourself into what was expected.

And somewhere along the way, you forgot how to hear the wild.

But she didn't forget you.

The System Benefits from Your Disconnection

Let's name what so few dare to say:

A wild woman is unmanageable.

She doesn't:

Fit into nine to five schedules.
Tolerate disrespect.
Swallow emotions to make others comfortable.
Buy what she doesn't need to impress people she doesn't trust.
Look outside herself for validation.
Silence her body's rhythms.

Which is why the system teaches you to:

Medicate your cycle.
Numb your intuition.
Suppress your anger.
Despise your body.
Obsess over productivity.
Apologise for taking up space.

Because when a woman remembers her wildness, She becomes sovereign. And sovereign women don't buy into systems that were built to break them.

What It Really Means to Rewild (And What It Doesn't)

Rewilding isn't just for those living in cabins, bleeding under the full moon, or growing herbs on a mountainside (though, goddess bless if that's your vibe).

Rewilding is a mindset.
A frequency.
A remembering.

It's about undoing the conditioning that told you you're only valuable when you're productive, presentable, or pleasing.

It's about coming back into a relationship with your instincts, your cycles, your land, your breath.

Rewilding is:

Screaming into the wind without guilt.
Saying no without explanation.
Eating when you're hungry, not when it's "time."
Resting when you bleed.
Walking barefoot on Earth just to feel her.
Letting your body guide your day, not your todo list.

It's not about perfection.
It's not about rejecting modern life.
It's not about performing a wild aesthetic for Instagram.

It's about reclaiming the parts of you that never belonged to the system in the first place.

The Sacred Power of Cycles

One of the biggest lies you were told? That you're meant to be the same every day.

Men live on a 24 hour hormonal cycle. The world was built for that rhythm, wake, work, perform, repeat.

But your body? Your body moves with the moon.

You are cyclical. You have inner seasons.
Your energy, focus, emotions, intuition, creativity, and libido shift throughout the month, and that is not weakness. It's wisdom.

Let's break it down:

Inner Winter (Menstruation)

- Time to rest, release, receive wisdom
- Your body wants stillness
- Deep intuitive clarity available if you slow down

Inner Spring (Follicular Phase)

- Energy returns
- Creativity flows
- Planning, preparing, and socialising feel natural

Inner Summer (Ovulation)

- Peak energy, magnetism, libido
- Great for outward expression, leadership, connection

Inner Autumn (Luteal Phase)

- Time to turn inward
- Deep discernment available

Moodiness often means misalignment is being revealed

When you ignore these seasons, you burn out.
When you honour them, you reclaim your power.

This is rewilding in action, living by the rhythm within you, not the rhythm imposed upon you.

Rewilding is Both Political and Personal

There's nothing neutral about a woman who listens to her body.

The moment you stop apologising for needing rest...
The moment you opt out of hustle culture...
The moment you cancel a plan because you're bleeding and need space...
The moment you speak your anger without softening it for others' comfort...

You are breaking invisible contracts.
Because we've been trained to override, smile, hustle, and perform.

Rewilding says: "I am no longer available for betrayal in the name of acceptance."

This isn't just self-care.
It's sacred activism.

And it begins with one yes to your wild self.

The Witch Wound & The Fear of Our Own Power

Let's call it what it is: we weren't just tamed, we were traumatised into forgetting our wildness.

For hundreds of years, women were tortured, burned, drowned, exiled, and publicly humiliated for doing things like:

Using herbs.
Bleeding with the moon.
Knowing too much.
Speaking too freely.
Being sexually free.
Being spiritually sovereign.

This wasn't just history.
It was a message.
A warning encoded into our bloodline.

"Stay small or you will not be safe."

Many of us carry this wound even now:

Fear of being seen
Fear of being misunderstood
Fear of judgment
Fear of being "too much"
Fear of saying the wrong thing
Fear of claiming our magic
Fear of being powerful in front of other women

This is the witch wound.

And rewilding?
It's not just about herbs and bare feet.
It's about healing this trauma so we stop betraying ourselves to stay safe.

Signs You've Been Domesticated

Most women don't even realise how much they've been conditioned until they try to break free.

Here are the signs of domestication:

You apologise for things you're not sorry for.
You hide your emotions, even from yourself.
You prioritise being liked over being honest.
You say yes when you mean no.
You dismiss your intuition as "silly" or "overthinking".
You feel guilty for resting.
You silence your truth to keep the peace.
You shapeshift to match the room you're in.
You judge other women for being too loud, too sexy, too spiritual, too wild.

It's not your fault.
This conditioning runs deep.
But the moment you notice it?
You're no longer bound by it.

Awareness is the first act of rebellion.

Daily Rewilding Practices (That Don't Require a Forest)

You don't need to abandon your life to rewild.
You don't need to move off-grid or throw out your phone (unless you want to).
You need to choose yourself, every day, in small, sacred ways.

Here are some modern rewilding rituals to begin with:

1. Let Your Body Lead

Move intuitively. Dance with your eyes closed. Let your hips guide you, not your head.

2. Bleed With Intention

Track your cycle. Mark it on your calendar. Rest when bleeding. Honour what's leaving your body. Journal during your luteal and menstruation phases.

3. Touch the Earth Daily

Even if you live in a flat, stand on the soil. Breathe the air. Talk to your plants. Let your feet touch something real.

4. Speak Without Softening

Say what you need without apologising first. Practice full sentences like: "No." and "I'm not available for that."

5. Unshame Your Pleasure

Touch your own body with reverence. Explore desire. Speak about sex like the sacred act it is.

6. Uncover the Cages

Ask daily: Am I doing this from truth, or from fear of not being accepted?

Reclaiming Instinct, Intuition, and Emotion

Wildness isn't chaos. It's clarity. It's the part of you that just knows.

When something isn't right
When someone isn't safe
When an opportunity is aligned

When your body needs to move, rest, cry, or scream

But for most of us? That knowing was buried beneath a lifetime of:

"Don't overreact."
"Don't be so sensitive."
"You're imagining it."
"Just calm down."
"You're being dramatic."

So we started second guessing ourselves.
We learned to ask others for permission to trust our own bodies.

We swallowed our grief, our rage, our joy.

But emotion is not weakness. Emotion is wild wisdom moving through flesh.

Your tears are sacred.
Your anger is a boundary enforcer.
Your fear is a messenger, not a jailer.
Your desire is divine.
Your grief is a midwife for rebirth.

You do not need to be less emotional. You need to feel it fully, move it wisely, and alchemise it fiercely.
That's rewilding.

Ritual: Earth, Blood & Breath

This ritual reconnects you to your primal wisdom, the part of you that never forgot.

You'll need:

- A private outdoor space or open window
- A small bowl of soil or salt
- Red thread or cloth (optional)
- Your breath

1. Sit or stand facing the Earth.
If outdoors, place your feet on the ground.
If indoors, hold your bowl of soil or salt in your lap.

2. Breathe deeply. In through the nose, out through the mouth.
Let the breath get deeper with each cycle. Let the wildness rise.

3. Place your hands on your womb or heart.
Say aloud:

*"I reclaim the wisdom of my body.
I reclaim the rhythm of my cycles.
I reclaim my sacred rage, my fierce joy, my primal softness.
I no longer apologise for the wildness in me.
I am not broken, I am blooming."*

4. Wrap the red thread around your wrist (or place the cloth in your altar space).

Let it be your reminder: you walk with the wild now.

Sacred Journal Prompts

Where in my life am I still playing small to stay safe?
What part of my wild feminine self have I hidden or silenced?
When was the last time I truly let myself feel, without censoring it?

What would it look like to trust my instincts again?
How can I honour my cycle, emotions, and sensuality in my daily life?

You Were Never Too Much. You Were Always Wild.

This chapter is not about becoming something new.
It's about remembering.

You were born wild.
You were taught to tame.
You were told that silence was safety.
You were told that softness was submission.
You were told that emotions were embarrassing.
You were told that power was dangerous.

But deep down, you always knew that the wild in you is holy.

Rewilding is the path back to that knowing. Not just for you, but for every woman who still believes she has to earn her worth.

Now you know better. Now you feel better.
And now?

You lead. Wild and sovereign.

CHAPTER 6

The Truth About Healing

Healing is not becoming a better version of you.
It's remembering who you were before the world told you to be anything else.

You likely came to healing the way most of us do.
Exhausted.
Frustrated.
Sick of quick fixes and temporary relief.
Ready for real change.

And somewhere deep down, you probably believed:

"If I just find the right practitioner, the right diet, the right supplement, the right moon phase, the right mindset... then I'll be okay. Then I'll be healed."

You imagined a moment where the pain would stop.
Where the symptoms would vanish.
Where your nervous system would settle for good.
Where life would finally feel light, aligned, easy.

But here's the truth:

Healing isn't a linear checklist.
It's not a one-time destination.
It's not a straight path from pain to perfection.

Healing is cyclical.
Messy.
Sacred.
Relational.
And almost never looks the way you expected.

The Healing Fantasy

Let's be real. At some point, we've all fallen into the fantasy:

You start a new protocol and believe, "This is it."
You finally quit gluten and wait for the enlightenment to hit.
You invest in a course, a coach, a cleanse, convinced this is the one.
You light the candle, pull the cards, drink the herbs, meditate… and then life punches you in the womb.

It's not that those tools aren't powerful. They are.
It's that we've been conditioned to chase healing like it's a product.

We treat healing like it should follow Amazon Prime rules: Click. Purchase. Transform in 2-5 working days.

But healing is not a product. It's a process. A deeply personal, often invisible, wildly nonlinear spiral back to truth.

Healing Is Not Linear

The linear model looks like this:

Start in pain → do the work → arrive in peace → live happily ever after

But in reality? It's more like:

Start in pain → do the work → feel worse → want to quit → have a breakthrough → feel amazing → crash again → question everything → rest → rise → repeat

And that is normal.

The spiral isn't failure.
It's the nervous system learning safety.

It's your cells unravelling trauma.
It's your ego learning to soften.
It's your soul remembering how to come home.

Every descent holds a teaching.
Every flare-up holds a message.
Every backslide is an initiation.

You're Not Doing It Wrong

Let's just say this now for the version of you who needs to hear it:

If you're crying more, you're not broken.
If you're exhausted, you're not failing.
If you're feeling more before you feel better, you're on the exact path.

Because true healing is not about feeling good all the time.
It's about becoming safe enough to feel what was never allowed before.

That's the truth they don't put on wellness packaging.

But it's the truth that sets you free.

Why It Gets Worse Before It Gets Better

Here's a truth most people won't admit, especially in the curated world of healing influencers and polished morning routine videos:

Healing hurts before it helps.
Because real healing isn't surface level.
It's deep tissue excavation.
It's nervous system reprogramming.
It's calling back every part of you that got locked away when it wasn't safe to feel.

And when you begin that process?
The body remembers.
The pain resurfaces.
The old coping mechanisms scream.
The trauma you thought was "dealt with" rises like smoke.

Your ego panics.
Your mind spirals.
Your nervous system flares.
And suddenly, you're wondering:
"Why the hell did I ever start this?"

But here's what you need to know:

This is the fire of transformation, not failure.

This is your body trusting you enough to reveal what was buried. This is healing, in its most raw and sacred form.

The Nervous System and the "Push-Back" Effect

Let's talk about your nervous system, because if you don't understand this, you'll keep interpreting progress as regression.

When you begin healing, whether it's through detoxing, resting, changing relationships, confronting your past, or regulating your cycle, you disrupt your nervous system's familiar pattern.

And even if that pattern was toxic, chaotic, or harmful… it was predictable.

So when you try to shift it?

Your nervous system sounds the alarm:

"Unfamiliar = unsafe."

Cue:

Panic attacks you haven't had in years.
Old symptoms flaring.
Relationship tension rising.
Dreams filled with grief or confusion.

Doubt crawling back in, louder than ever.

This is called resistance.
It's not your fault. It's biology.
Your system is testing whether the new path is truly safe.

And your job? To stay. To breathe. To anchor in the truth that what's surfacing is not a sign to stop, it's a sign to keep going.

How to Know If It's Resistance or Intuition

"But what if this is my intuition telling me to stop?"

Excellent question. Here's how you can tell the difference:

Intuition whispers. Resistance yells.
Intuition feels like a truth you already knew.
Resistance feels like a fear dressed as logic.
Trust your body to tell the difference.

Don't Abandon Yourself When the Spiral Hits

This is where most people quit.
Right here.
In the messy middle.
When it feels like nothing's working.

The Sacred Rebellion

When the new way feels impossible and the old way still calls your name.

They abandon the work.
Abandon their bodies.
Abandon the tools.
Abandon their truth.

Not because they're weak. Because they were never shown what the spiral of healing really looks like.

But now you know.
And that means you can choose differently.

You can stay.
You can soften.
You can breathe through the discomfort.
You can remind yourself: "This is the part where I rise."

Because it is.

The Healing Spiral

Forget the idea of a straight path.
Forget the fantasy of once-and-done healing.

Because healing doesn't happen in a line.

It happens in a spiral.

You return to the same wounds, but from a higher level of awareness.
You revisit the same emotions, but with more capacity.
You face the same patterns, but with more tools, more boundaries, more self-love.

It's not that the pain never leaves.
It's that you're no longer the same person facing it.

Think of it like this:

The Spiral Looks Like:

Grieving the same thing again, but crying less and feeling deeper. Getting triggered by the same situation, but recovering faster. Falling into old patterns, but catching yourself sooner. Revisiting trauma, but choosing to stay present instead of dissociating. Feeling fear, but not letting it make your choices anymore. This is progress.
This is healing. This is the spiral.

It doesn't mean you're back at square one. It means you're spiralling upward through layers, each round offering more truth, more release, more liberation.

Real-Life Healing Spiral Examples

Example One: Burnout

Round one: You crash and burn after ignoring your body for months.
Round two: You recognise the warning signs but still push through, then crash again.
Round three: You feel the first signals and choose rest early. You don't crash. You integrate.

That's not weakness. That's embodiment.

Example Two: Relationship Patterns

Round one: You attract emotionally unavailable partners and don't notice until you're heartbroken.
Round two: You notice red flags earlier but ignore them.
Round three: You walk away the first time your boundaries are violated and you don't need drama to justify it.

That's not being cold. That's healed discernment.

Example Three: Chronic Symptoms

Round one: You panic every time your symptoms flare, spiralling into fear.

Round two: You still flare, but now you respond with support, rest, herbs, presence.
Round three: You notice what triggered the flare and adjust before it escalates.

That's not failure. That's body trust.

What Healing Actually Feels Like

Let's normalise the truth.

Healing often feels like:

Deep grief with no clear source
Massive fatigue after emotional breakthroughs
Rage toward people who benefited from your silence
A sudden inability to tolerate anything misaligned
Feeling like a stranger in your own life
Losing friends, habits, beliefs, and entire identities

Because when you change your frequency, your life must recalibrate.

It's not that healing breaks things.
It reveals what was already broken underneath your coping mechanisms.

And from there?
You get to rebuild. Real. Rooted. Raw.

Signs You're Healing (Even If It Doesn't Feel Like It)

Healing isn't always fireworks and milestones.
Sometimes, it's subtle. Soft. Invisible to everyone but you.
It's in the tiny pivots. The internal shifts. The moments no one claps for.

Here's what healing actually looks like:

You feel anxious… but you don't run. You sit. You breathe. You stay.
You notice tension in your jaw and release it, instead of pushing through.
You crave sugar or a hit of dopamine, but you pause and check in before acting.
You speak your needs, even though your voice shakes.
You rest without guilt (or with slightly less guilt than before).
You make a choice that honours your energy, not your ego.
You realise you're tired and cancel a plan, without explaining yourself to death.
You stop explaining yourself at all.
You notice your triggers but no longer collapse into them.
You celebrate your wins, even the quiet ones.

That is healing. And every time you notice one of those moments? Mark it. Honour it. That's your proof. That's your spiral rising.

The Medicine of Going Slowly

You've been conditioned to rush.
To get to the destination.
To "fix" fast.
To make your body shut up so you can get on with life.

But healing is a relationship. And like all relationships, it thrives in presence, not pressure.

The truth?

Slower healing lasts longer.
It doesn't collapse under stress.
It integrates. It anchors. It holds.
It becomes your new baseline, not just a high from a temporary breakthrough.

Let your progress feel like a slow exhale.
Let your breakthroughs feel like gentle waves.
Let your rebirth come in layers, not explosions.

That's real. That's embodied. That's sustainable.

Daily Anchors for Sustainable Transformation

Healing doesn't happen in massive overhauls.
It happens in repeatable, doable daily practices that honour your body's needs and your soul's truth.

Here are a few powerful anchors:

1. Ground First, Then Act

Before reacting, deciding, responding, breathe into your body.
Ask: "Is this my truth or my trauma talking?"

2. Track Your Wins

Keep a notebook or notes app.
Each day, jot down one moment you responded differently.
Call it: The Spiral Journal.

3. Choose One Nervous System Ritual a Day

Examples:

- 3 minutes of humming or vagal toning.
- 1-minute cold face plunge.
- Barefoot on Earth.
- Hand on heart, eyes closed, deep breaths.

- Swapping your to-do list for a "to-be" list.

4. Honour Your Energy Cycles

Don't force productivity during your luteal phase or bleed.
Build your life around your body, not the other way around.

5. Speak Gently to Yourself

If your inner dialogue wouldn't nurture a child or a plant, rewrite it.
Daily mantra: "I trust the pace of my healing."

These aren't tasks. They're love letters to the version of you that's already arriving.

Ritual: Spiral of Healing Embodiment

This ritual honours the spiral you're walking, messy, sacred, and yours.
You'll need:

- A quiet space to stand or move
- A candle (optional)
- A piece of paper + pen
- A small object to represent your current self (a stone, shell, crystal, etc.)

The Sacred Rebellion

1. Stand in the centre of your space.
Visualise a spiral beneath you, winding inward and outward.

2. Begin slowly walking in a spiral.
Start from the outside. With each step, whisper something you've survived. A pain. A pattern. A lie you've released.

As you walk closer to the centre, whisper:

"I am still here."
"I am rising."
"I am remembering."

3. When you reach the centre, pause.
Place the object down. This is you now. Not perfect. Not finished. Just true.

4. Write on the paper:

"I honour the spiral.
I choose slow, sovereign healing.
I trust the return to my truest self."

Burn the paper (safely), bury it, or fold it into your altar.
You have marked your rebirth.

Sacred Journal Prompts

What is one thing I believed about healing that I'm ready to release?
How does my body let me know that I'm growing, even when my mind resists?
What does "healed" actually mean to me? How does it feel, smell, move, look?
Where in my life am I rushing? What would soften look like here?
What is one small ritual I can commit to daily, not for perfection, but for presence?

You Are the Healer You've Been Waiting For

Here's the wild truth:

There is no final arrival.
No healed version of you that floats through life untouched by pain or challenge.

There is only this:
Your return to yourself.
Layer by layer.
Breath by breath.
Spiral by spiral.

You will forget. And you will remember.

You will fall. And you will rise.

But now you know...
You don't need to be fixed.
You need to be felt.
You need to be heard.
You need to be held, by you.

That is the truth about healing.
Not the fantasy.
But the freedom.

CHAPTER 7

Detoxing the Mind, Spirit & Soul

Not all toxins live in your bloodstream. Some live in your thoughts. Your lineage. Your aura. Your memory. Your silence.

You've cleared your cupboards. You've swapped your skincare. You've learned to trust your symptoms, your cycles, your body.

But there's still heaviness. Still fog. Still inner chaos.

Because physical detox is only one layer. The most invisible, insidious toxins don't live in your kitchen. They live in your mind, your spirit, and your soul.

The belief that you're never doing enough.
The inner critic that echoes a parent's voice.
The soul contract to carry everyone's pain.
The fear that speaking your truth will cost you love.

The energetic cords that drain you before you even wake up.

This is the weight you were never meant to carry. This is the toxicity you won't find on a label and this is where your next level of healing begins.

What Spiritual Detox Actually Means

Let's get this straight, spiritual detox isn't just about burning sage, cutting cords, or taking salt baths under the full moon (though we love those too).

Spiritual detox means releasing the invisible attachments that cloud your mind, drain your life force, and keep you looped in patterns that don't reflect your truth.

It's not about becoming "pure."
It's about becoming free.

This kind of detox includes:

Thoughts you inherited that were never yours
Energy you absorb from people, places, and pain
Karmic patterns running in the background of your life
Inner voices that sound like you but belong to someone else
Guilt, shame, or fear that don't match your current reality

This is the detox no one sees.
But it shifts everything.

Mental Clutter: The Thoughts That Keep You Sick

Your body hears everything your mind says.

And if your internal dialogue sounds like:

"I'll never get better."
"I'm too much."
"This is just how I am."
"I can't trust myself."
"If I speak up, I'll lose love."
"I always mess things up."
"I don't deserve to rest."
"Healing works for others, but not for me…"

…then you are living in a toxic thought field, one you didn't consciously choose, but one you must now clear.

These beliefs create:

Nervous system dysregulation.
Chronic stress responses.
Hormonal imbalances.
Low energetic frequency.

Resistance to healing modalities.
Sabotage in relationships, work, and even healing itself.

This isn't spiritual fluff. This is neuroscience, epigenetics, and energetic hygiene all rolled into one.

Your Mind is a Garden, Not a Battlefield

You're not here to control every thought. That's impossible.
You're here to become conscious of what thoughts take root.

Ask yourself daily:

Is this thought mine?
Does this belief help me expand, or does it shrink me?
Would I speak to someone I love the way I'm speaking to myself?

You don't need to silence your mind.
You need to cleanse it.
With truth.
With compassion.
With clarity.
With sacred boundaries between you and the noise.

The Soul Toxins We Don't Talk About

Not every burden you carry is yours.
Not every voice in your head is your truth.
Not every ache in your body is from this lifetime.

Some wounds are ancestral.
Some patterns are energetic.
Some trauma is karmic.
And some contracts were formed in survival, not sovereignty.

This is the deeper detox. The kind that happens in the spirit, not the stomach. The kind that breaks soul cycles, not just surface habits.

Let's name what needs clearing:

1. Energetic Attachments & Parasites

Yes, this is real, and no, it's not always dramatic or demonic.

An energetic parasite is any entity, thought form, or attachment that feeds off your life force without your conscious permission.

You may notice:

Persistent fatigue despite physical healing.

Intrusive thoughts or sudden mood shifts.
Feeling "not yourself" in certain places or after certain interactions.
Regularly attracting draining, chaotic, or manipulative people.
Feeling watched, unsettled, or "open" even in sacred space.

These aren't always entities in the horror movie sense. Sometimes, they're leftover cords from past relationships. Sometimes, they're thought forms built from years of shame or fear. Sometimes, they're ancestral wounds being replayed through your energy body.

And they're not here because you're weak. They're here because your light is powerful. Which means… you have full authority to clear them.

2. Old Soul Contracts & Vows

You may have made unconscious spiritual agreements in this life, or past ones.

Vows like:

"I must carry everyone's pain to feel loved."
"I will never be powerful again because it wasn't safe last time."
"I must suffer to be spiritual."
"If I heal, I'll lose connection with my lineage."

"It's safer to stay small."
These aren't just ideas. They're energetic bindings and until they're revoked, they shape your patterns.

But here's the good news. You can rewrite them. You can declare new contracts from your healed self.

3. Karmic Debris & Lineage Inheritance

Some heaviness you carry didn't begin with you.

You may be the first in your family to seek healing.
The first to say no.
The first to rest.
The first to break cycles of control, codependency, or silence.

That means you're not just healing for yourself. You're transmuting generations of suppression.

You may feel:

Guilt when things get easier.
Grief that isn't yours.
Responsibility to carry others.
Fear of being different from your family.
Pressure to "fix" what you didn't cause.

Let me be clear:
You are not here to carry it all.
You are here to end it with love.

And that requires clearing what was never yours to begin with.

The Thought Patterns Blocking Your Healing

Some thoughts are just noise. But some are programs, repeating code embedded in your consciousness.

These mental patterns act like energetic malware.
They drain your light.
Distort your intuition.
Keep you loyal to versions of yourself you've long outgrown.

Here are some of the biggest mental toxins and their antidotes:

Toxic Thought: "I'm too much."

Spiritual Detox: You are not too much, you are too true for a system built on suppression.

Toxic Thought: "If I change, they'll leave."

Spiritual Detox: If your evolution threatens their presence, they were never meant to witness your becoming.

Toxic Thought: "I should be over this by now."

Spiritual Detox: You're not late, you're in rhythm with your soul's spiral.

Toxic Thought: "I must be doing something wrong if I'm still struggling."

Spiritual Detox: Progress doesn't always look like peace. Sometimes it looks like truth rising from the ashes.

These thoughts aren't just inconvenient.
They are anchors to your old self.
They whisper your fear back to life.
They convince you to play small under the guise of "being realistic."

But now that you can see them clearly, you get to choose again.
And this time? You choose freedom.

How Energetic Clutter Creates Spiritual Resistance

You can be doing everything right physically and still feel stuck.

Because if your energy field is filled with:

Old contracts.
Leaky boundaries.
Residual cords.
Karmic guilt.
Ancestral obligation.
People-pleasing masks.
Shame loops.

Then it doesn't matter how clean your diet is. Your soul is still clogged.

Energetic clutter can feel like:

Chronic indecision.
Restlessness with no root.
Feeling "off" for no reason.
Difficulty meditating or grounding.
Receiving intuitive hits, but second-guessing them constantly.
Being spiritually gifted, but afraid to use your power.

You are not blocked, you're buried. You don't need to be fixed, you need to be freed.

This is where deep soul detox begins.

Preparing for Conscious Sovereignty

You are no longer here to be a sponge for collective pain. You are here to become a clear, sovereign, sacred vessel.

That means:

Ending energetic contracts that drain you.
Releasing roles that were never yours.
Declaring what is no longer welcome in your field.
Calling your power back home.
Remembering that your energy is not charity, it is currency.

From now on, your aura is a temple and not everything gets to enter.

Shadow Work Is Energetic Alchemy

You can't spiritually detox without meeting your shadow.

Not because your shadow is bad or broken. But because everything you avoid becomes a toxin in your system.

What is shadow work?

It's the process of facing the parts of you you've hidden, denied, or rejected.
It's:

The unexpressed rage.
The hunger for validation.
The jealousy you shame.
The grief you suppress.
The desires you silence.
The power you're afraid to own.

And when those parts are pushed into the dark, they don't disappear.

They manifest as:

Chronic symptoms.
Emotional volatility.
Energetic leaks.
Sabotage cycles.
Depression, numbness, or fatigue.
Attraction to toxic relationships or spiritual bypassing.

Shadow work isn't easy. But it's liberating.

Because when you integrate your shadow? You take your power back. You stop leaking energy to suppression. You become whole again.

Protection vs. Armouring

You don't need to protect your energy by becoming cold, closed, or hard. That's not sovereignty, that's fear in fancy clothes.

You can be open-hearted and energetically boundaried.
You can be compassionate without being a sponge.
You can say no without guilt.
You can clear your field without cutting yourself off from love.

Energetic Boundaries That Don't Harden Your Heart

Start your day with a grounding visualisation: "I am rooted. I am sealed. I am sovereign."

Create a mental image of your aura, golden, fluid, and discerning. Speak this before entering any space: "Only love and truth may enter my field."

After intense conversations or crowds, do a clearing sweep with your hand or sacred smoke.

If you feel heavy, pause. Breathe. Ask: "Is this mine?" If not, return to sender with love.

You're not weak for feeling everything. You're powerful for not letting everything in.

Daily Detox Practices for Mind, Spirit & Soul

This isn't about rituals that take hours or require a mountain retreat. It's about sacred consistency. A few minutes a day that change your frequency.

Here are some potent practices:

1. Energetic Shower Releasing
As you wash, speak aloud: *"I release what is not mine. I release what no longer serves. I call all my energy back now."*

2. Morning Aura Activation
Sit for 3 minutes. Breathe. Visualise golden light around your body. Say: "I am light. I am clear. I am protected. I am me."

3. Journal Dump & Burn
Write the thoughts looping in your mind, no filter. Burn or rip the paper. Let it go physically and energetically.

4. Breath + Sound Release

Inhale deep. Exhale with sound. Hiss, sigh, hum, moan, or growl, whatever your body needs to release.

5. "Cord Check"

At the end of each day, ask:
Who am I still entangled with?
Who is still living in my thoughts?
Who do I need to cut cords with gently tonight?

Then, visualise it: a soft severing, a thank you, and a release.

You are your own energetic sanctuary. These practices are how you clean the altar of your spirit.

Ritual: Cord Cutting & Light Reclamation

This ritual clears energetic residue and calls your soul fragments home.

You'll need:

- A quiet space
- A candle (white or black)
- A piece of string or thread
- Scissors

Optional: sage, incense, or your favourite clearing herb.

1. Prepare your space.
Light the candle. Sit with your spine upright.
Breathe into your belly until you feel settled.

2. Take the string and hold it between your hands.
Visualise someone or something you're still entangled with.
An ex. An old identity. A trauma. A fear. A contract.

Say aloud:

"I honour the role this has played in my journey. But I am no longer bound to it.
With love and clarity, I release this tie.
I reclaim my light. I reclaim my space. I reclaim my soul."

3. Cut the string.
Watch the separation. Breathe.
Let your shoulders drop. Let your field expand.

4. Optional: Pass the smoke of sage or incense over your body.
Visualise your aura sealing in gold light.

Say: *"I walk forward clear, whole, and sovereign. I carry only what is mine."*

Blow out the candle. Drink water. Ground.
You've just cleared an old life from your field.

Sacred Journal Prompts

What energies, beliefs, or stories am I ready to release for good?
Who or what have I been energetically tied to that no longer reflects who I am?
What does a mentally clear, soul-led version of me look and feel like?
Where has my energy been leaking and how will I reclaim it now?
What new contract am I ready to write with my spirit?

You Are Your Own Sanctuary

You don't need to be rescued.
You don't need to be cleared by someone more "spiritual."
You don't need to earn the right to feel whole.

You are the keeper of your own light.
You are the guardian of your energy.
You are the priestess of your soul.

This detox isn't about becoming "pure."
It's about becoming real.

You're no longer available for energetic clutter.
You're no longer hosting beliefs that shrink your truth.
You're no longer carrying karma that was never yours.

You are clear.
You are anchored.
You are walking your path fully awake, fully you.

And that?
That's the soul detox complete.

CHAPTER 8

Building a Life That Heals You

You weren't made to hustle through exhaustion. You were made to design a life that restores you every single day.

You've detoxed the products. You've cleared the energy. You've listened to your body, reclaimed your wildness, remembered your power.

And now? You build.

Because healing isn't just about what you release. It's about what you replace it with.

You can't heal inside the same environment that made you sick. You can't become your truest self while still living someone else's blueprint.

You came here to design a life that:

Supports your nervous system.
Matches your values.
Aligns with your cycles.
Expands your spirit.
Heals you as you live it.

This chapter is your invitation to do exactly that.

What It Means to Live in Healing Alignment

Healing alignment doesn't mean you never feel pain, stress, or fatigue. It means your default life rhythm supports your body, not battles it.

It means:

You stop glorifying burnout
You stop betraying your yes and no
You stop settling for chaos just because you're used to it

And instead:

You honour your energy flow.
You design your days around restoration.
You say yes only when your body also says yes.

You surround yourself with resonance, not obligation.
You live a life that feels like breathing, not performing.

That is what alignment feels like: ease, clarity, and deep breath returning to the system.

From Survival to Sacred Design

Most of us were never taught how to build a life. We were taught how to survive one.

Get a job that pays the bills.
Push through exhaustion.
Drink caffeine to keep going.
Rest only when you're broken.
Adapt to environments that harm you.
Make it look good, even if it feels like hell.

But that's not design. That's survival in a costume.

Now? You get to design something sacred. A life that fits your nervous system, your truth, your body, your soul.

This is more than lifestyle.
This is lifestyle as ritual.
As devotion.
As medicine.

Identifying What Drains You

Before you build a life that heals you, you must see, with raw honesty, what's currently keeping you unwell.

Some things are obviously toxic. Others are deceptively subtle. They mask themselves as "normal," "necessary," or "not that bad."

But here's the truth:

Anything that chronically contracts your body, dims your truth, or erodes your energy, is a drain.
And drains, left unaddressed, become disease.

Let's identify them now.

1. Draining People

These are not just "bad vibes" or energy vampires.

These are people who:

Expect access to you, but offer nothing in return.
Guilt you into connection.
Refuse to honour your boundaries.
Talk at you, never with you.

Leave you feeling smaller, tense, or tired after every interaction.

It could be a friend, a family member, a client, or even someone you love deeply. But if the energetic exchange is chronically one sided?

It is costing your health.

2. Draining Habits

These are behaviours that slowly chip away at your vitality:

Skipping meals or eating in stress.
Scrolling first thing in the morning.
Saying "yes" when your body says "no".
Going to bed wired and waking up exhausted.
Consuming content that triggers comparison or hopelessness.

These habits don't make you bad, they make you human in survival mode. But now you know better. Now you get to choose again.

3. Draining Environments

Yes, your physical space has a frequency.

Your nervous system responds to:

Clutter.
Fluorescent lights.
Constant noise.
Lack of nature.
Unfiltered technology.
Air filled with artificial scent and stagnant energy.

If your home, workspace, or even your car feels like it's squeezing you instead of supporting you, that is not "just life."

That is a call for recalibration.

4. Draining Obligations

The silent killers of life force:

"I should…"
"They expect me to…"
"I can't say no because…"
"It's just easier to go along with it…"

Every time you override your own truth to keep someone else comfortable, you lose a piece of your power.

Healing alignment means unlearning the lie that obligation is love, and remembering that your yes means nothing if your no isn't sacred.

Auditing Without Guilt

This is not about blame. It's not about throwing everything out and starting over.

It's about getting honest about what your body has known for a long time. And asking the question: "Is this costing me more than it's nourishing me?"

From that place of truth, we build something new.

Creating Rhythms That Regulate & Restore

You don't need a stricter routine. You need a softer rhythm.

Healing doesn't thrive in pressure.

It thrives in pattern. In familiarity. In daily rituals that say: "You're safe. I've got you. You don't have to brace anymore."

Your body is a rhythmic being:

Your heart beats in rhythm.
Your breath flows in rhythm.
Your hormones cycle in rhythm.
Your sleep, digestion, temperature, all tied to rhythm.

When life pulls you out of rhythm? Your body begins to dysregulate. You lose energy, clarity, emotional balance, and connection to self.

But when you restore rhythm, you restore safety.

Let's do that now.

Designing a Day That Heals You

Here's what a healing-aligned day might include.
Not as a checklist, but as an invitation:

Morning (Opening Ritual)

- Wake gently, no jolting alarms or instant screens.
- Hydrate your body.
- Light movement or stretching.
- Gratitude, breathwork, or intention-setting.
- A nourishing breakfast eaten without multitasking.

Why it matters: You're setting your nervous system's tone for the day. A regulated morning = more resilience to whatever follows.

Midday (Sustaining Ritual)

- Eat before you're starving
- Get outside, even for 5 minutes
- Body check-in: "What do I need right now?"
- Say no to something misaligned, just once
- Rest, not just when you crash, but before you reach depletion

Why it matters: You anchor into sovereign energy management, instead of riding chaos waves.

Evening (Closing Ritual)

- Put your phone away early (ideally 1–2 hours before sleep)
- Dim the lights
- Nourish your body again, even something small
- Journal, stretch, or use calming herbs/oils
- Offer gratitude, not because life was perfect, but because you showed up

Why it matters: You're signalling to your body: "It's safe to let go now."

Soul-Led Structure vs. Toxic Productivity

Structure is not the enemy.

Rigid structure = control
Soul-led structure = safety

Toxic productivity says:

"You can't rest until everything is done."
"If you slow down, you'll fall behind."
"Prove your worth through your output."

Soul led structure says:

"What would feel supportive today?"
"How can I honour my cycle and energy?"
"What can I let go of to protect my peace?"

One burns you out. The other builds you up.

Designing Your Environment for Nervous System Safety

Your nervous system doesn't only respond to thoughts and trauma. It responds to space. To light. To noise. To clutter. To the layout of your home.

You can regulate your body simply by adjusting your environment.

Let's get something straight:

Healing doesn't mean your home must be spotless, beige, and minimalist.

It means your space should feel like a soft exhale.
It should hold you. Not overstimulate you.
It should speak: "You're safe here."

The Frequency of Your Home

Every item you keep, every scent you use, every sound you allow into your space, carries frequency.

Ask yourself:

Does this space feel calming or chaotic?

Can I rest here without effort?
Do I feel at home here... or do I just live here?
What am I tolerating in my space that no longer reflects who I am?

Your home is an extension of your energy field. Clear your home, and you clear you.

The Subtle Energetics of Clutter

Clutter is more than an eyesore. It's energetic congestion.

It creates:

Mental fog.
Procrastination.
Shame spirals.
Stagnant chi.
Resistance to clarity, creativity, and healing.
But decluttering doesn't need to be overwhelming. It can be devotional.

Let every drawer you clear be a prayer.
Let every item you release be a spell: *"I make space for more of me."*

Clearing with Intention

1. One space at a time, even a single shelf is a win.

2. Ask each item:

Do I use this?
Do I love this?
Does this reflect the version of me I'm becoming?
3. Let go lovingly. Thank it. Release it.

4. Clean with herbs or oils: Lemon, rosemary, lavender, cedarwood, all clear stagnant energy.

5. Play music, light incense, open the windows. Make it sacred.

Sensory Sanctuaries

Your space should nourish your senses. Here's how to make that happen:

Sight

- Warm lighting over harsh white bulbs.
- Nature elements: plants, wood, stones.
- Visual inspiration that uplifts, not overwhelms.

Sound

- Lo-fi beats, nature sounds, silence over background TV.
- Avoid constant noise, it spikes cortisol.
- Sound bowls or bells to reset the energy.

Scent

- Natural essential oils: think lavender, peppermint, orange, eucalyptus.
- Avoid synthetic air fresheners and candles, they disrupt hormones.
- Smudge with intention (use ethical herbs or botanicals that honour the space).

Touch

- Soft blankets, natural fabrics, cozy corners.
- Let your space invite you into rest and softness.

Your space is either helping your body return to peace…
Or keeping it in quiet alert.

Let this be the moment you choose to build a healing nest.

Building a Circle That Heals, Not Drains

No one heals in isolation. But not every connection is healing.

As you shift, grow, and reclaim your truth, your circle will shift too.

Some will cheer.
Some will vanish.
Some will resist your change.

Let them.

You're not here to fit back into old roles.
You're here to build a support system that nourishes the healed version of you, not the wounded one.

What a Healing Circle Feels Like

You feel safe being messy.
Your boundaries are respected, not resented.
You're celebrated for your growth, not guilt tripped for it.
You don't have to dim your light to protect someone else's shadow.
You leave conversations full, not empty.

Healing circles don't need to be large. They need to be aligned.

You don't need more people. You need the right people.

Ritual: Crafting Your Sacred Life Blueprint

This ritual guides you into intentional design, choosing the life you want to live from the inside out.

You'll need:

- A journal or notebook
- 30 minutes of quiet
- A candle (optional)

Step 1: The Audit

Draw a line down the centre of your page.

Left side: What drains me?
Right side: What nourishes me?

Write without editing. Include people, habits, spaces, thoughts, responsibilities.

Step 2: The Vision

Write at the top of a new page: *"If my life was designed to heal me, it would look like..."*

Let it flow. Don't try to make it realistic. Make it true. Let your nervous system and soul write this with you.

Step 3: The Blueprint

Answer the following:

What will I stop tolerating in my space, time, and body?
What one rhythm, habit, or ritual am I ready to commit to now?
What environment will I create that reflects my healed self?
What does my sacred 'yes' feel like? My sacred 'no'?

This is your foundation.
This is your rebellion, in form.

Sacred Journal Prompts

Where in my life am I still living in survival instead of sovereignty?
What rhythms would my body create if it could lead my life?
Who in my life truly sees me, and who only sees the version they're comfortable with?
What would it feel like to rest inside my life, not just escape from it?
What kind of woman am I designing this life for?

This Is the Life You Came Here to Live

You are not here to recover from your own life.
You are here to build one that heals you in real-time.

A life that reflects your healing.
Holds your softness.
Honours your no.
Celebrates your yes.
And expands with you as you grow.

That life is not a fantasy.
It's a decision.
It's a blueprint.
And it begins with one sacred choice:

You no longer build from survival.
You build from sovereignty.
From softness.
From wild, anchored truth.

And that changes everything.

CHAPTER 9

Raising the Next Generation Free

You are not just healing for you. You are healing for every child who will never have to recover from your survival.

Let's get one thing clear from the start:

You do not have to be a parent to be a cycle-breaker.
You may be a mother, an aunt, a teacher, a mentor, a godparent, or a soul who simply chooses to do it differently, and that is enough.

Because every time you:

Say "I love you" without conditions.
Apologise when you mess up.
Regulate instead of react.
Validate instead of shame.

Listen instead of silence.

Choose presence over perfection...

You become the ancestor they don't have to heal from.

The Echo of Our Unhealed Lineage

Most of us were raised by people who were surviving.
Parents who loved us... but never learned how to love themselves.
Carers who meant well... but never had models for emotional safety.
Generations of adults who repeated what was done to them, and called it normal.

So we inherited:

Shutdowns instead of conversations.
Silence instead of apologies.
Fear-based discipline instead of mutual respect.
Emotional absence disguised as strength.
Conditioning to obey rather than express.

And from that soil, we grew roots that didn't feel safe to stay grounded in.

But now?

We get to compost all of that.
We get to turn the pain into wisdom.
We get to raise the next generation in liberated soil.

Why Healing Ourselves Is the Most Radical Parenting We'll Ever Do

You can read all the parenting books.
You can buy the wooden toys, the toxin-free weaning bowls, the Montessori shelves.
You can do every "right" thing.

But if your nervous system is dysregulated…
If your voice is full of unprocessed rage…
If your eyes carry grief that's never been named…
If your touch flinches before it soothes…

Your child will feel it.

Children don't learn from what we say.
They learn from what we embody.

If you honour your truth, they will honour theirs.
If you apologise when you're wrong, they'll feel safe to be human.
If you treat your body with reverence, they'll do the same.
If you validate emotions instead of managing them, they'll trust their own compass.

This is what it means to raise the next generation free: You model the freedom they'll one day claim as their birthright.

What Our Children Really Inherit (Beyond DNA)

When we think of inheritance, we think of eye colour. Height. The shape of their nose.

But what your children inherit goes far deeper than biology.

They inherit:

Your nervous system patterns.
Your emotional vocabulary.
Your relationship to truth.
Your beliefs about the body.
Your model of self-worth.
Your template for love, rest, and power.

This is not to shame you. This is to free you.

Because you are not doomed to repeat the past. You are the living pivot point.

They Inherit Your Regulation

Children don't regulate themselves.
They learn regulation through co-regulation, through your breath, tone, posture, presence.

If you scream when overwhelmed, they learn to panic.
If you shut down, they learn to disappear.
If you hold your breath under stress, they learn the world is not safe.

But...

If you breathe through the mess?
If you narrate your emotions instead of hiding them?
If you model rupture and repair?

They learn resilience.
They learn safety.
They learn how to meet life without abandoning themselves.

That's not small. That's legacy.

They Inherit Your Unspoken Beliefs

Even when you don't say it out loud, they feel it.
If you call yourself ugly in the mirror, they absorb self rejection. If you ignore your needs, they learn their needs are inconvenient.
If you stay silent to "keep the peace," they learn truth is dangerous.
If you hate your body, they learn to disconnect from theirs.
If you never rest, they learn rest is weakness.
If you apologise for your existence, they learn to shrink.

The deepest lessons are the ones we never knew we were teaching.

And that means the greatest healing begins when you stop asking, "What do I need to teach my child?"

and start asking,
"What do I still need to learn, feel, and reparent in myself?"

From Control to Conscious Connection

Many of us were parented through control.

"Because I said so."
"I'm the adult."
"You don't get a choice."
"Stop crying or I'll give you something to cry about."

We were trained to obey, not to trust. To please, not to express. To survive, not to thrive.

But conscious connection means:

You guide, not dictate.
You listen, not dismiss.
You explain, not manipulate.
You honour their sovereignty, not override it to prove your authority.

It doesn't mean you let chaos rule. It means your power comes from relationship, not force.

And when your child feels respected, heard, and safe?
They don't need to rebel to find freedom.
They already live in it.

Reclaiming Sacred Discipline (Without Punishment)

Let's be clear, discipline and punishment are not the same thing.

Punishment is rooted in control, fear, shame, and power imbalance. Discipline, when practiced consciously, is an act of guidance and devotion.

It doesn't say, "You are bad."

It says, "This is the impact of your actions, and I love you enough to hold you through the repair."

Discipline Becomes Sacred When

It focuses on connection before correction.
It teaches cause and effect, not right and wrong.
It holds firm boundaries with softness.
It models emotional accountability, not blame.
It invites reflection, not repression.
It keeps your child's dignity intact.

You can be both loving and firm.
You can hold space for their emotion and guide their behaviour.
You can uphold boundaries without breaking their spirit.

This is not permissive parenting. This is reverent leadership.

And it builds children who trust you, and themselves.

Teaching Body Wisdom and Sovereignty from the Start

You don't need to wait until your child is a teenager to talk about consent, intuition, and boundaries.

They start learning those things from birth, through how you treat their body, respond to their signals, and honour their voice.

Body Wisdom Is Taught When You:

Ask permission before hugging or tickling

Let them say no, even to adults.
Teach them the names of their body parts without shame.
Encourage rest, food, and movement based on how they feel.
Help them tune into emotions in their belly, chest, throat, etc.
Trust their no, even when it's inconvenient.

When a child is raised to listen to their body, they don't grow up needing someone else to translate its wisdom for them.

That's the foundation of sovereignty.

Creating Homes That Regulate, Not Overstimulate

You don't need Pinterest perfection. You need a space that feels safe to feel.

Children thrive in:

Predictable rhythms.
Soft lighting and sounds.

Space to move and be loud.
Places to retreat and be quiet.

Homes where they're not "too much" for the adults around them

Your home doesn't need to look like a magazine.
It needs to feel like a nervous system sanctuary.

That means:

Less "stuff," more space to breathe.
Less overstimulation, more connection.
Less chaos, more rhythm.
Let your home say: "You are welcome here exactly as you are."

Raising the Sensitive, the Neurodivergent, and the Soul Led

Some children won't fit the systems. Not because something is wrong with them. But because their blueprint was never meant to submit.

They come in highly sensitive.
Neurodivergent.
Multidimensional.
Soul led.

They come in:

- Feeling everything
- Asking big questions
- Struggling with rigid routines
- Thriving in freedom, but melting in control
- Needing slowness, softness, space, and permission to be exactly who they are

And here's the truth most won't say:

These children are not broken.
They are oracles in tiny bodies.
And they are here to break the system, not be broken by it.

What They Need Isn't Perfection. It's Presence.

You don't need to have all the answers.
You don't need to fix everything.
You don't need to "normalize" them.

You need to:

Co-regulate when they unravel.
Learn their rhythms instead of forcing your own.
Protect their energy, not just their bodies.
Speak to their soul with honesty and respect.

Teach them that being different isn't a defect, it's a design.

When a sensitive child is honoured, they become an intuitive adult.
When a neurodivergent child is supported, they become a genius in their own lane.

You are not raising conformity.
You are raising liberation in motion.

Ritual: The Ancestral Line Ends With Me

This ritual marks the point of transformation, the place where cycles of control, suppression, shame, and survival end with you.

You'll need:

- A bowl of water or earth
- A candle
- A photo or symbol of your lineage (optional)
- A quiet space

1. Light your candle.

Say aloud: *"I honour the ones who came before.*
I acknowledge the pain passed through generations.
I witness it. I hold it. I choose to end it."

2. Place your hands in the bowl of water or on the earth.

Say: *"I return the burdens that were never mine.*
I release the pain that does not belong in the future.
I bless the line forward, with truth, with love, with freedom."

3. Place your hand on your heart.

Speak this truth into your bones: *"The line ends with me.*
The line heals with me.
The next generation will be free."

Blow out the candle. Breathe. You just rewrote the future.

Sacred Journal Prompts

What patterns am I refusing to pass on?
What does a free child look like, sound like, and feel like in my world?
Where do I still parent myself from punishment instead of compassion?
What new beliefs am I planting in my family line today?
What kind of ancestor am I becoming?

You Are the Turning Point

Your children don't need you to be perfect. They need you to be brave.

Brave enough to:

Break silence
Hold space
Say no to traditions that harmed you
Build new ones rooted in truth
Honour what's hard and keep going anyway

You may never get thanked.
You may never see the full fruits of your healing.

But one day, a child will sit in their wholeness and wonder, "How did I get so free?"

And the answer will be:
Because someone before me chose to heal.
Because someone loved me enough to stop the cycle.
Because someone chose to remember.
Because someone... was you.

Chapter 10

Sovereignty as a Lifestyle

Healing got you here. Sovereignty takes you home.

There comes a moment in every healing journey where you realise…

You don't need another detox.
You don't need another course.
You don't need another guru, book, protocol, or permission slip.

You just need to choose yourself.
Loudly. Quietly. Consistently.
In every space, every season, and every version of you.

That moment?
That is the birth of sovereignty.

Freedom vs. Sovereignty

Let's clear something up.

Freedom is the ability to choose. Sovereignty is the ability to lead yourself through those choices, with clarity, consistency, and inner truth.

Freedom says, "I don't want to be controlled."
Sovereignty says, "I am the one I trust to guide me."

Freedom is a taste. Sovereignty is a practice.

Freedom is the first rebellion. Sovereignty is what you build in the ashes.

Sovereignty Is Not a Mood. It's a Lifestyle.

You're not sovereign when you're having a great day.

You're sovereign when:

Your boundaries are tested, and you honour them anyway.
You're triggered, and you don't outsource your power.
You're unsure, but still move from truth.

The world says "go left" and your body says "go right" and you listen.

Sovereignty is not loud. It's not about dominating others or being hyper-independent.

It's a quiet knowing that you are your own authority. And you don't need to prove it to anyone.

Why Sovereignty Starts in the Body

You cannot be sovereign in your life if you are disconnected from your body.

Because sovereignty requires sensation.
Presence. A deep-rooted "yes" or "no" that comes from your cells, not your logic.

It's why every system that seeks to control people, especially women, starts by disconnecting them from their:

- Intuition
- Cycles
- Desires
- Sensuality
- Gut instincts
- Nervous system regulation

But you've reclaimed that now.
You've remembered how to listen.
And that makes you unstoppable.

Because when a woman is in her body. She's in her power. And when she's in her power? She becomes sovereign.

Detoxing People Pleasing, Perfectionism, and Performance

You can detox the products. You can detox the pharmaceuticals. But if you're still addicted to approval?

You're not free.

If you still:

- Say yes out of guilt
- Stay quiet to avoid judgment
- Perform a version of yourself that others can digest
- Shape shift to stay accepted
- Apologise for taking up space

Dull your truth so no one feels uncomfortable…

Then your sovereignty is still on pause. Let's call these behaviours what they are: survival strategies. They were formed in childhood to help you feel safe, loved, and accepted.

But now? They're just holding you back.

People Pleasing

Looks like kindness. Feels like self-erasure. You're not choosing connection, you're avoiding rejection.

Perfectionism

Looks like high standards. Feels like chronic tension. You're not seeking excellence, you're trying to avoid punishment.

Performing

Looks like charisma. Feels like exhaustion. You're not expressing, you're editing yourself to be palatable.

These aren't flaws. They're invitations. Every time you catch yourself people pleasing, perfecting, or performing, ask:

"What part of me is still afraid I won't be loved if I'm fully seen?"

And then remind her:
You are worthy, even when you're messy.
Even when you're real.
Especially then.

Anchoring Into Sacred Values

Sovereignty isn't about control. It's about clarity.

When you know what truly matters to you. You stop chasing what doesn't.

So let's bring this home.

What Are Sacred Values?

They are the pillars you build your life around.
They are your compass when the world gets noisy.
They are the boundaries you enforce, not out of ego, but out of honour.

Examples:

- Peace over performance
- Truth over comfort
- Depth over small talk
- Integrity over popularity

- Rest over hustle
- Expression over suppression
- Connection over convenience
- Body wisdom over external rules

You don't just declare your values once. You live them daily.

When you know your values, decisions get easier and when your life reflects them, you feel safe, because you're in alignment.

Reclaiming Your Time, Energy, and Decisions

If your time belongs to everyone else, if your calendar is filled with shoulds, if your energy is leaking through silent obligations and unchecked notifications...

Then you're not living sovereignly, you're managing yourself like a resource for others.

Sovereignty says: I get to decide. Not in rebellion from responsibility, but in deep reverence for your capacity, your desires, and your nervous system.

You reclaim your time when you...

Start your day on your terms (not in reaction to messages or demands).

Block out sacred space for your own rituals, even if it's 10 minutes.
Say "not right now" without apology.
Recognise that urgency is rarely sacred, and rest is not optional.

You reclaim your energy when you...

Tune into what drains you (and take action to shift it).
Honour your cyclical nature, not override it.
Spend time with people who nourish, not deplete.
Make space to do nothing and be still without guilt.

You reclaim your decision making power when you...

Trust your gut and act on it.
Let your values, not validation, guide your yes and no.
Stop waiting for someone else to give you permission.

Know that if it costs your peace, your truth, or your alignment...
It's too expensive.

Creating Systems That Serve You

Let's be real, sovereignty doesn't mean chaos.
It means building systems that serve you, not the other way around.

You get to choose:

What time your day starts.
How many hours you work.
What kind of movement supports your body.
Which rituals ground and guide you.
What kind of boundaries honour your energy.
When to walk away, when to show up, and when to completely unplug.

And if that doesn't fit the matrix? Even better.
This is your rebellion in practice, daily, gentle, and radical.

Walking Through the World as a Sovereign Woman

She doesn't walk faster to match the world's pace.
She doesn't water herself down to be digestible.
She doesn't explain her boundaries.
She embodies them.

She doesn't need a crown to be recognised. She is the crown.

A sovereign woman doesn't just do different, she is different.

Her presence feels like truth.
Her energy feels like permission.
She's magnetic, not because she's loud, but because she's aligned.

She Knows...

Her body is her compass.
Her rest is her right.
Her boundaries are sacred altars.
Her decisions are hers to make.
Her yes is full-bodied.
Her no is non-negotiable.

She doesn't seek approval. She walks with self authority.

She's not afraid to take up space. She's afraid of shrinking ever again.

Rewriting Identity from Wholeness, Not Wounding

When you've built your identity around pain, you feel unanchored when it begins to heal.

Who are you if you're no longer the fixer, the martyr, the overachiever, the wounded one?

You are free. You are whole.

And now... you get to write a new story.

Not from survival.

Not from performance.
But from sacred, embodied truth.

You are not who they told you to be. You are not even who you had to be. You are who you choose to become. That is sovereignty.

Ritual: The Crown Returns

You'll need:

- A candle
- A mirror
- A space to stand or sit with presence
- Optional: a physical crown, flower halo, scarf, or symbol

1. Light the candle. Face the mirror. Breathe.

Say aloud:

*"I no longer abandon myself to be accepted.
I no longer outsource my truth.
I reclaim my power now."*

2. Place your crown or symbol onto your head. Close your eyes. Visualise a golden light rising from the earth and descending from the stars, meeting at your crown.

Say:

*"My sovereignty is sacred.
My choices are mine.
My body is wise.
I walk in wholeness now."*

3. Stand tall. Say your name. Say it again.
Speak it like a spell.
Because it is.

Journal Prompts

Where in my life have I outsourced my truth to feel safe or accepted?
What does a sovereign 'yes' feel like in my body? A sovereign 'no'?
What systems in my life need to change so that they serve me, not control me?
Who am I when I am no longer living from wounds, roles, or expectations?
What does walking in wholeness look like for me, every day?

You Are the Authority Now

You are no longer waiting for someone to tell you what's right. You are no longer asking for permission to slow down, speak up, or walk away. You are no longer living in fragments.

The Sacred Rebellion

You are whole.
You are wise.
You are sovereign.

And from here forward, everything you create will carry the frequency of a woman who knows herself.

This is not the end of your healing. It's the beginning of your reign.

CHAPTER 11

The Separation Myth: How Disconnection Fuels Disease

You were never meant to live in boxes.
Drive through concrete jungles.
Sit under fluorescent lights.
Stare at screens for hours while your bare feet never touch the soil.

And yet, this is the world many of us were raised in.

Disconnected from the sun, the moon, the land, and our own bodies.
Taught to fear dirt, silence, and stillness.
Taught that the Earth was something to be used, not known.

This is the first wound.

We were severed from the source that created us. Then shamed for why we're sick, anxious, inflamed, and exhausted.

Disconnection Is a Design

It's no accident that our systems teach us to ignore:

- Hunger cues
- Sleep cycles
- Menstrual rhythms
- Emotional waves
- Seasons of rest

Our connection to the land and living beings around us.

Because when we forget our place in nature. We forget our power.

We become easier to manipulate.
Easier to sell to.
Easier to medicate, numb, and control.

But the Earth Never Forgot You

While you've been aching for rest.
She's been whispering in winds and rivers.
Calling you back in every sunrise.
Waiting for you in the scent of the forest floor.

Holding your rage in storm clouds.
Cradling your grief in the ocean's tide.

She remembers.
She remembers who you were before the world told you to perform.
She remembers the version of you that wasn't disconnected.
Just buried.

The Cure Begins at the Root

This chapter isn't about sustainability trends or outdoor aesthetics. It's about sacred reconnection.

It's about reclaiming your birthright as a living, breathing extension of the Earth. Because when you return to her, you return to you.

Rewilding the Body and Soul

You weren't born to be tame. You were born to be whole. And wholeness includes the wild.

But somewhere along the way, your instincts were labelled too much. Your intuition was ignored. Your cyclical nature was shamed and your wildness was called unruly.

This wasn't by accident. It was conditioning.

Domestication is Disconnection in Disguise

From an early age, we are trained to:

Sit still when our bodies want to move.
Be quiet when our emotions want to roar.
Smile when we want to scream.
Follow rules that ignore our rhythm.
Abandon our inner truth for outer validation.

This is the beginning of soul amnesia.

We forget what we once knew:

That our bodies are sacred instruments, not machines.
That our emotions are messengers, not disruptions.
That our sensitivity is a superpower, not a flaw.
That the Earth is our mirror, not our backdrop.

To Rewild Is To Return

Rewilding isn't about moving into the forest and foraging herbs by moonlight (although, if that's your vibe, yes, please).

It's about:

Moving your body in ways that feel instinctual, not performative.
Listening to your hunger, rest, and emotional cues without shame.
Bleeding, crying, or raging without apology.
Taking off the mask and remembering the animal inside your skin.
Letting nature remind you who you are when you're not performing.

Rewilding is sacred remembering.

It's you, barefoot in the grass.
Body humming with truth.
Heart unfiltered.
Breath deep and untamed.
No longer asking the world for permission to exist in your natural state.

You don't need to be fixed.
You need to be returned.

Back to the Earth.
Back to your rhythm.
Back to the version of you who was never broken.

Returning to the Rhythms of Nature

Nature doesn't rush. She doesn't hustle. She blooms, rests, dies, and rises again, on purpose, with purpose.

And you, dear one, were made of the same rhythm.

But the modern world will have you believe:

You're lazy if you rest.
You're behind if you're not producing.
You're unwell if you're cycling through emotions.
You're broken if you're not always "on".

This isn't truth. It's programming and the Earth is here to unteach it.

The Rhythm of the Seasons Lives in You

Just like the Earth, you move in seasons:

Spring – The rise, the renewal, the inspired momentum.
Summer – The radiance, the action, the outward expression.
Autumn – The letting go, the harvest, the sacred slowing.
Winter – The rest, the retreat, the quiet integration.

You are not meant to be in a perpetual summer.

You are not a machine. You are cyclical. And your body will begin to heal when it is allowed to move like the Earth does, with rhythm, not resistance.

The Wheel of the Year: Ancient Rhythms Remembered

For those who follow Earth-based traditions, the year was always understood as a wheel, not a straight line.

Each sabbat, solstice, and equinox reflected not only what was happening in the land but also what was happening within.

- Imbolc (Feb 1–2): New ideas stirring under the surface
- Ostara (Spring Equinox): Balance and blooming
- Beltane (May 1): Fire, fertility, and full-bodied living
- Litha (Summer Solstice): Peak power and light
- Lammas (Aug 1): Gratitude and gathering
- Mabon (Autumn Equinox): Release and reflection
- Samhain (Oct 31–Nov 1): Death, ancestors, shadow
- Yule (Winter Solstice): Stillness and sacred rebirth

These were not just festivals. They were soul mirrors.

And when we return to them, We return to timing that honours our humanity.

Healing Through Seasonal Alignment

When you align your energy, work, rest, rituals, and healing with the Earth's rhythms, everything softens. The shame drops. The guilt lifts. The body breathes.

You stop trying to bloom all year. And instead, you root deep, rest well, rise strong, and let life live through you.

This is seasonal sovereignty.
This is sacred timing.
This is your body's natural pace, remembered.

The Earth as Mirror, Mother, and Memory Keeper

There's a reason you cry in the forest. Breathe deeper at the ocean. Feel something ancient stir when your bare feet touch the ground

The Earth doesn't just nourish you. She reflects you.

Every part of nature mirrors a part of your internal world:

Storms mirror your grief and rage.
Sunlight mirrors your joy and clarity.
Roots mirror your stability and depth.
Winds mirror your shifts and restlessness.
Waves mirror your emotions, fluid, powerful, rhythmic.

When you sit with her long enough,
You stop asking, "What's wrong with me?"
And start whispering, "Oh... this is just a season."

The Earth Remembers What You Forgot

She remembers when you danced without shame.
When you howled instead of swallowed your pain.
When you knew rest was sacred, not earned.
When you trusted your gut more than any guru.
When your rituals were instinct, not calendar reminders.

She holds all of it.

Every version of you that disconnected.
Every truth you silenced.
Every ancestral wound you inherited.
Every soul contract you came here to break.

It's all stored.
In the soil.
In the wind.
In the water.

And when you return to her, with presence, with humility, with bare feet and an open heart. She starts returning you to yourself.

She Is Not Just Land, She Is Legacy

The Earth is not just where you live. She is how you live.

She is where your ancestors bled, birthed, broke, prayed.
She is where your future generations will build, plant, and rise.
And in between? She is where you remember that you are not separate.

You are part of a sacred ecosystem. Your healing is her healing. Your liberation ripples through the mycelium, the soil, the skies.

The Earth is not outside of you. She is beneath you, within you, around you, and always waiting for you to come home.

Elemental Healing: Fire, Water, Earth, Air, Spirit

The elements are not symbolic. They're alive and they've been waiting for you to return.

When the world gets too loud,
When your body feels like a stranger,
When your healing feels like too much to carry.

Come back to the elements.
They know what to do with everything you're holding.

Fire: The Alchemist

Fire is the sacred destroyer and the holy igniter.
She burns what no longer serves.
She brings light to the dark.
She creates heat, movement, and momentum.

Call on fire when:

You need to let go of a belief, behaviour, or identity.
You're ready to activate courage and forward movement.
You want to transform grief, rage, or stagnation into sacred fuel.

Practice:
Burn a written belief you're shedding.
Dance wildly by candlelight.
Let your anger move through you like wildfire, then watch what grows after.

Water: The Healer

Water doesn't ask you to explain.
She just holds you while you feel.

She flows. She cleanses. She softens the sharp edges.

Call on water when:

You feel emotionally blocked, brittle, or overwhelmed.
You need to cry, release, or be soothed.
You want to remember how to flow instead of fight.

Practice:

Take a ritual bath with herbs or salt.
Cry into a river or rainstorm.
Drink water with intention, asking it to heal from the inside out.

Earth: The Root

Earth is your anchor. Your stillness. Your stability.
She holds your weight without judgement.
She reminds you that presence is power.

Call on earth when:

You feel ungrounded, anxious, or disconnected.
You need to rebuild trust in your body and instincts.
You're calling in safety, nourishment, and slow, sustainable healing.

Practice:

Lay on the ground and feel your heartbeat return to the soil.
Walk barefoot on natural earth.
Place your hands in dirt, clay, or sand and let the earth speak through sensation.

Air: The Breath of Clarity

Air is your voice, your perspective, your mind in motion.
She cuts through confusion. She whispers truth.
She invites you to expand.

Call on air when:

You feel foggy, creatively blocked, or mentally cluttered.
You're ready to speak something out loud that's been buried.
You want to shift your inner story or self-perception.

Practice:

Breathe deeply and audibly. Let it be a release.
Speak your truth into the wind.
Write a new belief and read it aloud beneath the sky.

Spirit: The Remembering

Spirit isn't above the elements, it's within them. It's the thread that connects fire to water, earth to air, body to soul. It is the part of you that has never forgotten why you're here.

Call on spirit when:

You want to reconnect to your inner guidance.
You're ready to co-create with something higher.
You desire to remember that your healing is a sacred path, not a checklist.

Practice:

Sit in silence and ask, "What do I need to remember?"
Pull an oracle card and meditate on the message.
Speak your name aloud as a sacred invocation.

You don't need a certification to work with the elements.
You only need presence.
And willingness.
They already know what you've come for.

Let them meet you there.

Sacred Reciprocity: Living in Right Relationship

The Earth gives without asking for praise.
She gives you air, food, medicine, beauty, and shelter.
And yet most of us were never taught how to give back.

We take.
We extract.
We consume.
And then we wonder why we feel disconnected.
Right relationship is the medicine.
Reciprocity is the realignment.

Healing Isn't Just Personal, It's Planetary

You cannot separate your own healing from the Earth's.

When you:

Clean your body of toxins.
You reduce what flows back into the soil and water.
When you regulate your nervous system.
You stop passing down trauma to the next generation.
When you choose slow, handmade, intentional living.
You break the spell of extraction culture.
You become the rebellion.

You move from consumer to steward.
From What can I get? to How can I honour this exchange?

Ways to Practice Sacred Reciprocity

You don't need to own land or start a homestead to live in sacred exchange with the Earth.

Start with presence. Then...

Give offerings – herbs, flowers, words, prayers, or your bare hands in the soil.
Listen more than you speak – nature always answers, but you must get quiet to hear her.
Tend, don't just take – plant something. Restore something. Return something.
Live with reverence – from the way you source your food to the way you dispose of waste.
Ask before you harvest – and say thank you every time you do.
Support the protectors – those defending water, land, and indigenous knowledge need our voices and our action.

This Isn't About Perfection. It's About Intention.

You're not expected to live waste-free, barefoot, and growing your own kale by moonlight (unless you want to).

But you are being invited to remember.
That the Earth is alive.
That she responds to your energy.
That she recognises when you walk through the world with reverence.

Reciprocity is a frequency and the more you live in it, the more whole you will feel.

Soil, Soul, and Sovereignty

You weren't meant to heal in a vacuum. You weren't meant to chase freedom on digital timelines alone. Your sovereignty is not only about your choices. It's about your roots.

And the Earth is where you plant them.

Why the Land Matters

We've been told our healing is individual. That it lives in affirmations and apps, in talk therapy and self-care routines.

But healing is also land-based.

Your nervous system doesn't just crave safety. It craves belonging.

The Earth gives you that. The soil holds it. And your sovereignty is activated when you stop floating and start rooting.

Land is Legacy

The land holds your ancestors' footsteps, even if they were displaced. It holds the medicine of your lineage, even if it was stolen, suppressed, or silenced.

And when you reconnect to land, whether it's your ancestral soil or the earth beneath your current feet.

You begin to reclaim something deeper than knowledge.
You reclaim memory.
You reclaim purpose.
You remember that your body is not separate from the soil, it is soil.

Sovereignty Begins in the Ground Beneath You

When you root into land (even in a small garden, a potted plant, a community allotment, or simply barefoot in the grass), you reclaim your place in a lineage that predates capitalism, colonialism, and control.

You remember:

You are cyclical like the seasons.
You are wild like the weather.
You are sacred like the soil.
You are enough like the seed.
And you belong here.

Ritual: Root to Remember

You'll need:

- A patch of earth (or a pot of soil if indoors)
- A small offering (flower, herb, crystal, or prayer)
- Your bare feet or hands

1. Stand or kneel with your body touching the soil.
Place your hands or feet on the ground. Close your eyes.
Breathe into your body until you feel heavy, in a good way.

Say aloud:

*"I root into the Earth that remembers me.
I return to the land that holds me.
I release the illusion of separation."*

2. Offer your gift to the land.
Place it into the soil with care. Whisper:
"Thank you for holding what I forgot. I remember now."

3. Stay in silence.
Let the Earth speak back. Through sensation. Through emotion. Through stillness.
You may not hear words, but you will feel something shift.

Journal Prompts

What parts of me feel most disconnected from the Earth, and why?
What do I remember about myself when I sit in nature?
Where can I begin practicing sacred reciprocity in my life right now?
What does it mean to live in right relationship, with the land, with my body, with my soul?
If my soul were soil, what would it need to feel nourished?

Grounding Integration

You don't have to move to the mountains or disappear into a forest to return to the Earth.

You only have to slow down.
Take off your shoes.

Put your hands in something real.
And remember that you are not separate.

The Earth is not just the ground beneath your feet.
She is your mirror.
Your memory.
Your mother.
Your medicine.
And she has been waiting for you to come home.

Chapter 12

The War on the Body: Cultural, Systemic, Personal

Let's call it what it is: You were born into a world at war with your body.

And that war has many names:

- Diet culture
- Medical gaslighting
- Purity culture
- Fatphobia
- Beauty standards
- Disability bias
- Productivity obsession
- Pharmaceutical dependency

You've been taught that your body is a project to be fixed. A problem to be solved. A thing to shrink, silence, sculpt, suppress, sedate.

You were never taught to trust it.

The Body Was Never the Problem

When you had a symptom, they told you it was random.
When you had a need, they called you high maintenance.
When you spoke your pain, they told you it was in your head.
When you tried to rest, they called you lazy.

But your body? It was always speaking truth. It just never spoke the language they wanted to hear.

Systems Thrive When You Distrust Yourself

When you disconnect from your body, you:

Spend more to look the way you "should".
Take more to feel the way you "should".
Do more to keep up with what others are doing.
Hand over authority to anyone with a title or white coat.

This isn't just personal, it's systemic.

Because a woman who trusts her body is hard to manipulate.

A person who listens to their gut is dangerous to systems built on compliance.

A body in its full, unapologetic expression is a threat to every system that profits off your shame.

And Yet, Despite It All...

Your body has kept breathing.
Kept beating.
Kept whispering.

Through symptoms. Through exhaustion. Through shutdown and flares. It never gave up on you.

Now it's time to stop fighting it. And start coming home.

This chapter is about that return. To trust. To truth. To your own sacred body, awake, alive, and whole.

Symptoms as Signals, Not Failures

What if your pain wasn't a punishment?
What if your fatigue wasn't laziness?
What if your flare ups weren't betrayal, but a breakthrough trying to get your attention?

We're taught to fear symptoms. To silence them. To mask them. To medicate them into submission before we ever ask, "Why is this happening?".

But your body doesn't speak in words. It speaks in sensation. It speaks in patterns. It speaks in discomfort, because you've been taught to ignore the whispers.

And when you ignore the whispers? The body starts to scream.

Your Body Has Always Been Speaking

That lump in your throat?
That tightness in your chest?
That ache in your lower back that flares up when you're around certain people?

It's not random.
It's not weakness.
It's not "all in your head."

It's intelligence.
It's insight.
It's your body saying, Something here is not safe. Something here is not aligned. Something here needs your love and attention.

You Were Never Meant to "Fix" Yourself

The culture of optimisation tells you to:

- Biohack it
- Numb it
- Push through it
- Erase the evidence of your humanity
- Present as fine even when you're breaking

But healing doesn't always look like "getting better." Sometimes it looks like finally hearing your body's message. Even if the message is hard. Even if it disrupts everything you thought you knew.

Your goal is not to make the pain disappear at any cost.
Your goal is to learn its language.

Only then can true healing begin.

From Silence to Sovereignty

When you start interpreting your symptoms as sacred signals:

You move from fear to curiosity.
You stop fighting your body and start partnering with it.
You recognise that pain isn't the problem, it's the portal.

And that portal leads you somewhere deep. Somewhere wise. Somewhere only you can access.

Your body has been waiting for you to listen. This is you... tuning in.

Reclaiming Sensation, Pleasure, and Presence

You weren't born disconnected. You were born curious, sensory, expressive, wild. You reached for softness. You giggled at sunshine. You danced without choreography. You felt everything.

But over time... you were taught to numb. To ignore. To stay "in control."

Especially if you were a woman. Especially if you were sensitive. Especially if you were in pain.

Sensation became dangerous. Pleasure became shameful. Presence became uncomfortable.

But those things are your birthright.

Numbness Isn't Neutrality

Numbness might feel safe, but it's not sovereignty. It's survival.

You can't selectively numb. When you shut down pain, you also shut down joy. When you avoid discomfort, you also avoid ecstasy.

And I don't just mean sexual pleasure (although that's part of it). I mean the pleasure of being alive. The pleasure of deep breaths. Warm tea. Bare feet on cold ground. Laughter in your belly. Sunlight on your face. Quiet that settles in your bones.

Your body is wired for that. But it needs safety to access it.

You Can't Heal a Body You're Not In

Presence is the foundation of embodiment and embodiment is the foundation of healing.

If you're constantly:

- Distracting
- Pushing through
- Overriding cues
- Stuck in your head
- Feeling "floaty" or checked out

...your body doesn't feel safe. Not because it's broken but because it hasn't been listened to.

To reclaim sensation is to whisper to your nervous system: *"I'm here now. I'm listening. You're safe to feel again."*

Start With Micro-Presence

Coming back to your body doesn't have to be dramatic.

You don't need to meditate for hours or do ecstatic dance under the full moon (though go for it if it calls you).

Sometimes it looks like:

- Pressing your palm to your heart and breathing.
- Feeling the weight of your body in a chair.
- Noticing your breath during a conversation.
- Checking in before you say yes.
- Washing your hands slowly, letting the water anchor you.

These are sacred acts..These are how you come home. Not all at once. But one sensation at a time.

Pleasure is your portal. Presence is your power. And sensation is your body's way of saying, "I trust you again."

The Nervous System as a Spiritual Path

You can't override a dysregulated nervous system with positive affirmations. You can't manifest your way into safety if your body still feels under threat. You can't fully heal when you're still stuck in survival.

But here's the truth: Your nervous system isn't broken. It's brilliant. It's adaptive. It has been working tirelessly to keep you safe in a world that hasn't always been safe for you.

Understanding Your Body's Inner Compass

Your nervous system is the bridge between your body, your mind, and your spirit. It interprets the world for you. It shapes your sense of reality.

Through polyvagal theory, we understand that the nervous system responds to perceived safety and threat in three primary states:

1. Ventral Vagal – Safe, social, regulated.
2. Sympathetic – Fight or flight, mobilised, agitated.
3. Dorsal Vagal – Freeze, shutdown, numbness.

None of these states are wrong. They're all intelligent responses to your environment and past experiences.

You didn't "fail" by dissociating.
You didn't "fail" by getting stuck in anxiety.
Your body found a way to survive.

Spirituality That Doesn't Honour the Nervous System is Bypassing

If a healing modality tells you to "just let it go," "just raise your vibe," or "choose love over fear", but doesn't address your nervous system...

It's skipping over the most sacred part of your healing.

Because you can't ascend if your body still thinks it's under attack. You can't be present with your intuition if your brain is in survival mode. You can't "be the light" if your body is frozen in trauma.

Safety isn't soft, it's sacred.

Regulation Is Revolution

Regulating your nervous system is not just about staying calm.

It's about:

Expanding your capacity for sensation.

Being able to hold space for your emotions without dissociating. Feeling safe in your skin, even when the world feels unsafe. Reclaiming agency over how you respond, not just react.

This is embodied rebellion. This is where your healing becomes cellular.

When your nervous system is regulated, your body becomes a safe place to live again. And from that place? You don't just survive, you create.

Embodiment Practices That Actually Work

Let's be honest. The word embodiment gets thrown around like it's a lifestyle trend. But it's not about curated rituals or aesthetic yoga flows.

Embodiment is the act of staying in your body. When everything around you is trying to pull you out of it.

It's not about being calm 24/7. It's about being present, even in the storm. It's about staying with your breath, even when your mind wants to run. It's about feeling without abandoning yourself.

Your Body Doesn't Want Performance. It Wants Presence

The most powerful embodiment practices are the ones you can return to daily. You don't need candles, music, or perfect leggings. You need you.

Here Are Practices That Actually Work:

1. Orienting
Look around your space slowly.
Let your eyes land on something you like.
Breathe.
This tells your nervous system, *"We're not under threat. We can be here."*

2. Somatic Check-In
Ask: Where am I holding tension?
What am I feeling in my belly?
Is my jaw clenched?
What would soften me right now?

No fixing, just noticing.

3. Grounding Through Movement
Move your body like you're listening to it.

Let it guide you. No choreography.
Even swaying for 30 seconds is embodiment.

4. Tactile Anchoring
Press your hands to your heart.
Massage your temples.
Hold your own face.
Place a warm compress on your womb.
Let your body feel held, by you.

5. Embodied Breath
Not shallow. Not forced.
Just full, present, intentional.

Try this:
Inhale slowly for 4 counts.
Hold for 4.
Exhale for 6.
Repeat until you feel your body begin to settle.

It's Not What You Do, It's How You Do It

You can wash dishes in dissociation. Or you can wash them as an act of embodied presence. Same task. Different intention. Entirely different nervous system response.
Let your day become your practice.
Let your body become your altar.

Let each moment become your reclamation.
You don't need more steps. You need more presence.

And you're already enough to offer it.

Moving From Shame to Sovereignty

If you've ever looked in the mirror and felt disgust.
If you've ever apologised for your body taking up space.
If you've ever felt like your symptoms made you "less than".
If you've ever carried the weight of a diagnosis like a scarlet letter.

You are not alone.
And you are not broken.
You are sacred.

But shame... Shame makes you forget.

Shame Is a Control Strategy

Shame is not just an emotion, it's a system. It disconnects you from your body so that you'll control it, silence it, hide it, starve it, push it harder.

Shame tells you:

"Your pain is inconvenient"

"Your needs are a burden"
"Your belly is wrong"
"Your energy is too much or not enough"
"You should be more like her"
"You need to prove you're worthy of love, rest, or softness"

It doesn't matter if it came from family, religion, society, media, or medicine.

What matters is that it ends here.

Sovereignty Says: I Choose What This Body Means

Sovereignty doesn't mean loving your body every day. It means owning your body story. It means not letting shame be the author anymore. It means defining your worth on your own terms.

It means looking at a scar and seeing survival.
Looking at your belly and seeing wisdom.
Looking at your stretch marks and seeing softness.
Looking at your flare-ups and saying, "I will not abandon you."

Sovereignty says:

"I get to rest without guilt."
"I get to eat without punishment."
"I get to live fully, even if I'm not 'healed.'"

"I get to exist unapologetically, even in a body that's still learning how to feel safe."

You Are Not Your Diagnosis. Your Trauma. Your Size. Your Symptoms.

You are a soul. In a body. That has carried more than it should have. And it's still here. Still breathing. Still trying. Still waiting for you to say:

"I see you. I'm not leaving. Let's rise together."

Ritual – Listen to the Body Oracle

You'll need:

- A quiet space
- A journal
- Your hands
- A mirror (optional)
- An open heart and an hour to come home to yourself

1. Ground Yourself
Sit or lie down in stillness. Place your hands somewhere meaningful, your heart, belly, womb, or throat.
Breathe slowly, three times.

Let your awareness settle into your body, not your thoughts, not your timeline. Your body.

Say aloud:
"I am listening now."

2. Ask and Receive
Ask your body one of the following:
"What do you want me to know today?"
"What have you been holding in silence?"
"What do you need more of, less of, or to be released from?"

Then wait.

Don't force answers.
Let sensations, emotions, or images arise.
Don't judge what comes, just witness it.

3. Write the Message
Open your journal. Begin with:
"My body says…"
"My body needs…"
"My body remembers…"

Let it flow. Let it be messy. Let it be honest.

4. Mirror & Speak (optional but powerful)
Look into a mirror. Eye to eye. Soul to soul.

Say aloud:
"I see you."
"I trust you."
"You do not need to perform to be worthy."
"You are sacred."
"You are home."

Let the tears come if they do.
Let the voice tremble if it must.
You are remembering. You are rewriting.

Journal Prompts

What have I been taught to believe about my body that I now reject?
How does my body ask for rest, nourishment, or connection and how do I respond?
Where in my body do I feel the most disconnected? The most at home?
If I treated my body as sacred, what would change in my day-to-day life?
What do I need to say to my body right now?

Somatic Integration Suggestions

Walk slowly in nature while tuning in to each step.
Place one hand over your heart, one over your womb, and hum softly.
Practice shaking, release stuck energy through gentle, intuitive movement.
Speak a daily affirmation that isn't about looks or worthiness, but about trusting your body's truth.

You Are the Body. You Are the Oracle.

Your body is not something to escape. It is not something to fix. It is not something to apologise for. It is the living altar of your wisdom, your lineage, and your rebellion. Every stretch mark is a signature. Every scar is a story. Every breath is a blessing.

This isn't just a body. It's you, awake, alive, returning.

Chapter 13

The Addiction to Healing: When Healing Becomes a Cage

Let's get honest.

Healing is sacred. Healing is necessary. Healing can save lives. But healing can also become a trap.

The Healing Hustle Is Real

We're living in a culture where self development has become just another performance.

Where healing is:

Another thing to perfect. Another reason to delay joy. Another way to stay in a loop of never being enough.

You journal, meditate, reparent, shadow work, EFT tap, trauma track, energy clear, regulate your nervous system, cleanse your aura and somehow, it still doesn't feel like you've arrived.

Because somewhere along the way, healing became another form of self-surveillance. Another impossible standard. Another cage dressed up in spiritual language.

When Healing Becomes Self Abandonment

You start to believe:

"I can't have that relationship until I'm more healed."
"I can't launch that offering until I'm fully confident."
"I can't rest until I've earned it through progress."
"I can't be loved until I've fixed all my triggers."

But that's not healing. That's perfectionism in disguise. And perfectionism will always steal your joy and call it progress.

You Are Not a Constant Project

You are not broken glass to be glued together for someone else's comfort. You are not here to graduate from your humanity. You are here to live.

And healing? Healing is meant to return you to life. Not delay it. Healing is the doorway. Living is the point.

Integration as the True Medicine

Healing isn't about how many breakthroughs you've had.
It's about how deeply you're able to live what you've learned.

You don't need another lightbulb moment.
You need anchoring.
You need embodiment.
You need integration.

Integration Is the Sacred Pause After the Breakthrough

After the realisation…
After the ceremony…
After the therapy session…
After the workshop or trauma-informed post or ah-ha moment…

Your soul doesn't ask you to keep chasing. It asks you to rest. To digest. To make space for the truth to settle into your cells.

This is where real transformation happens.

Not when you know better. But when you live different.

Let Life Be the Practice

Integration is when you:

Say no without explaining and survive the silence.
Rest on a weekday without guilt.
Communicate a boundary without collapsing into shame.
Feed yourself well even when no one's watching.
Respond to a trigger with breath instead of backlash.
Choose presence over performance.

You won't always get it "right." That's not the point. Integration isn't perfection. It's repetition with grace.

You've Healed Enough to Live

This might be the scariest truth of all:
You've healed enough to live.

To love.
To lead.
To show up.
To take up space.
To begin.
To rest.
To stop working on yourself long enough to actually enjoy yourself.

You can keep healing, yes. But not at the cost of your aliveness. You do not need to wait until you're more whole, to be wildly, messily, sacredly alive. You are already worthy of your sacred life.

Devotion Over Discipline: Sacred Living in Action

You've been taught to chase routine like it's salvation. To master your morning. To hustle for your habits. To dominate your day with willpower and productivity.

But what if sacred living wasn't about control? What if it was about connection?

Discipline Says: "Do it or you're failing."
Devotion whispers: "Come home to yourself again and again."
One is rooted in fear. The other in love. One demands. The other invites. This is the difference between spiritual burnout and soul nourishment.

Devotion Doesn't Require Perfection

It doesn't care if you missed a day.
It doesn't punish you when you're tired.
It doesn't count your steps or scold your softness.

Devotion is how you make tea with presence.
How you tend to your altar, even when it's messy.
How you take your supplements with gratitude instead of guilt.
How you speak gently to yourself when old patterns flare.
Devotion is choosing again. Without shame. Without rules.
Without needing to earn your own tenderness.

Create Rhythms That Meet You Where You Are

Sacred living doesn't mean copying someone else's rituals.
It means finding what honours you.

Ask yourself:

What anchors me into my body?
What softens my nervous system?
What brings me closer to the Divine, to the Earth, to myself?
What rituals feel like love, not pressure?

Then do those things.
Consistently.

Lovingly.
Devotedly.

Discipline is loud.
Devotion is magnetic.
One will burn you out.
The other will bring you home.

Creating a Life That Doesn't Require Escape

If you're always waiting for the next retreat, the next holiday, the next weekend, the next scroll, sip, or sleep to feel okay...

Then the life you're living isn't in alignment. It's in survival. You weren't born to endure your own life. You were born to live it fully.

Escape Isn't the Problem, It's the Alarm

Everyone needs rest. Everyone needs spaciousness. Everyone needs a break.

But when your life becomes something you constantly need to escape from,
It's not a sign you're lazy.
It's not a flaw in your character.

It's a sacred signal.

A sign that something is off. That the structure of your days is out of resonance with your soul.

And you get to change that.

Build a Life That Feeds You Instead of Depletes You

Ask yourself:

What kind of life would I not need to recover from?
What would it feel like to wake up without dread?
What would change if my body, business, home, or relationships were built for sustainability, not just survival?

It doesn't have to be radical overnight.
It starts with tiny sacred shifts:

Swapping hustle for honouring.
Swapping constant doing for meaningful being.
Swapping "should"s for "soul says".

Design for Your Nervous System, Not Your Ego

A sacred life doesn't always look successful from the outside.
But it feels safe, aligned, and true on the inside.

That's the goal.

You don't need a life that impresses strangers. You need a life that lets you breathe deeply, love fully, and return home to yourself every damn day.
You are allowed to design a life
you don't want to run from.

That is sacred rebellion. And it's available to you now.

Embodying Your Medicine in the World

You don't need a certification to be a healer. You don't need 10,000 followers to be impactful. You don't need to "arrive" before you begin.

Your medicine is how you live.
How you love.
How you hold space.
How you speak truth.
How you walk into a room with a regulated nervous system and don't try to fix anyone.

That's powerful. That's rare. That's revolutionary.

You Are the Living Proof

Every boundary you hold with grace.
Every moment you choose presence over performance.
Every time you say no to burnout and yes to your body.
You are showing the world what healing looks like.

That is your medicine.

You don't have to teach it, preach it, or post it to prove it. You only have to live it.

Lead Without Rescuing

Your sacred life doesn't require you to be the hero.

You are not here to carry others across their own thresholds. You're here to light the torch and walk your own path so boldly that it gives others permission to do the same.

You are the lighthouse. Not the lifeboat.

You don't need to shrink, sacrifice, or save to be seen as spiritual.

You lead by being aligned. You guide by being grounded. You heal the collective by healing yourself, and living it out loud.

Your Embodiment Is Your Offering

No fancy funnels. No hustle. No polished perfection. Your embodied truth, your sacred life, your unfiltered energy, that's the work.
Whether you're parenting, painting, coaching, teaching, planting, serving, or simply being. Your frequency is felt. Your medicine is magnetic. And your presence is enough.

Embodying Your Medicine in the World

You don't need a degree to be a healer.
You don't need a perfect past to guide others.
You don't need to be 100% healed to be holy.

Your presence is medicine.
Your truth is a transmission.
Your embodiment is the revolution.

The World Doesn't Need More Experts It Needs More Embodied Leaders

We're not looking for people who've memorised the right words.
We're looking for those who live what they teach.
Who sit with their shadows and speak with compassion.
Who walk their talk, even if it's messy, slow, or unconventional.

Your story, raw and real, is a roadmap for someone else's return.

Don't Just Preach the Medicine, Be It

Being the medicine looks like:

Resting when your body asks, even when hustle whispers louder.
Speaking up when silence would feel safer.
Saying "I don't know yet" with humility instead of hiding.
Taking aligned action without seeking applause.
Choosing peace over performance.

You don't have to do it all. You just have to be true.

You Are Not the Lifeboat, You Are the Lighthouse

You are not here to save everyone. You are not here to drain yourself dry in service. You are not here to fix, rescue, or martyr your way into meaning.
You are here to shine. To anchor. To stand steady in your light.

And from that light, others find their way. Not because you pulled them through the storm, but because you reminded them they could survive it.

Embodying your medicine doesn't require effort. It requires alignment. And alignment comes when you stop trying to prove yourself... and simply live as yourself.

Ritual: Rise in Reverence

This is a ritual of becoming. Of anchoring the sacred self you've reclaimed, and choosing once and for all, to live from your soul, not your survival.

You'll need:

- A candle
- A mirror
- An item that symbolises your sacred life (jewellery, herb, stone, flower, crown)
- A quiet space

1. Light Your Flame
Let it be a representation of your own inner fire. As it flickers, whisper:
*"I am no longer healing to be enough.
I am enough, and so I live."*

2. Stand in the Mirror
Look into your own eyes. Let the silence settle. Place your chosen item on your body, your crown, your hand, your altar space.

Say aloud: *"I honour the body that carried me.*
I honour the pain that shaped me.
I honour the truth that awakened me.
And I honour the sacred life I now choose to live."

3. Speak Your Declaration
Complete this sentence aloud:

"From this moment forward, I choose a life that is..."

Let the words rise. Speak them as a spell. Write them down if you wish. Post them somewhere you'll see.

Let it become your mantra.

Journal Prompts

What beliefs about myself have I released during this journey?
What sacred truth have I reclaimed?
What does a sacred life look, feel, and move like for me?
How will I honour my truth even when the world forgets its own?
What will I create from this place of wholeness?

You are not just the reader.
You are the rebellion.
You are not a body in repair.
You are a sovereign soul in motion.

You are not a seeker.
You are a rememberer of what has always been true.

The Sacred Rebellion lives in your choices now. In your boundaries. In your softness. In your boldness. In your breath.

Let it echo in everything you touch.
Let it ripple through every generation to come.
Let it be known that you returned to yourself and rebuilt the world from that place.

You are the sacred.
You are the spark.
You are the revolution.

Live it well.
Live it true.
Live it loud.

YOUR JOURNEY CONTINUES HERE...

You've remembered. You've reclaimed. You've risen.

Now it's time to continue your sacred rebellion with the spaces, support, and soul nourishment that are here to hold you.

The Strange Apothecary

Where magic meets medicine.
Handmade, holistic, high vibration products designed to support your body, mind, and soul. From natural remedies to spiritual tools, each item is infused with purpose, potency, and planetary love.

Shop the revolution: strangeapothecary.co.uk

The Sacred Code Podcast

Where sacred chaos meets nervous system gold.
Welcome to *The Sacred Shi*tshow, hosted by Hannah Strange.
This isn't just a podcast. It's a reckoning. A regulation station.
A wild, witchy transmission for the brave hearts navigating healing, embodiment, and life's beautiful mess. Because being a whole damn human? That's the real spiritual rebellion.

Listen & subscribe: thesacredshitshow.co.uk

The Sacred Portal

The 5D healing experience your soul's been waiting for.

This isn't a course, it's a full-body, multidimensional rebirth. Move through ancestral wounds, energetic blocks, and the depths of your being in this 6 week guided experience with Hannah.
Because you weren't meant to heal alone, you were meant to return whole.

Join the portal: thesacredportal.co.uk

The Sacred Shitshow Membership

A sacred AF space for the soul-led, nervous system fried, and rebellion-fuelled. The Sacred Sh*tshow is a WhatsApp-based membership for women healing in real-time, no fluff, no filters, just tools, truth, and a whole lot of nervous system magic.

Expect daily regulation prompts, tarot with bite, real talk, live healing sessions, and a community that holds you through the chaos *without* expecting you to be "healed" first. It's messy. It's sacred. It's your next nervous system era.

Join the membership: thesacredshitshow.co.uk

Final Blessing

This isn't the end, love.
This is your beginning.

You don't need to ask permission to rise anymore. You don't need to wait for a better moment. You don't need to be more healed, more prepared, or more perfect.

You are ready.

The Sacred Rebellion is not just a book, it's a frequency. And you're now carrying it in your field.

Let it ripple.
Let it root.
Let it rise.

And when you forget who you are, return to these pages, to the earth, to your breath, and to the truth that never left you:

You were never broken.
You were born for this.

Acknowledgements

This book would not exist without the wild, wounded, and waking versions of me who refused to give up.

To my children, thank you for giving me purpose, presence, and fire.

To my sacred clients and community, you have taught me more than any textbook ever could.

To the ancestral and cosmic forces guiding this work, thank you for choosing me.

To those who doubted me, thank you for fuelling the rebellion.

And to the woman holding this book in her hands right now. Thank you for remembering who you are.

Resources

Books & Texts:

- *The Body Keeps the Score* by Bessel van der Kolk
- *Women Who Run With the Wolves* by Clarissa Pinkola Estés
- *Braiding Sweetgrass* by Robin Wall Kimmerer
- *Polyvagal Theory in Therapy* by Deb Dana
- *This is Your Brain on Birth Control* by Sarah E. Hill

Podcasts:

- *The Sacred Code Podcast* by Hannah Strange
- *On Being* by Krista Tippett
- *The Holistic Psychologist*

Websites & Tools:

- strangeapothecary.co.uk
- The Sacred Portal Healing Programme
- The Sacred Forest Membership
- Nervous System regulation resources from Deb Dana & Polyvagal Institute

Glossary of Sacred Terms

Ancestral Healing
The process of clearing inherited trauma, beliefs, and patterns passed down through your lineage. This work honours your ancestors while freeing future generations.

Cellular Healing
Deep, somatic-level transformation that affects not just your mind, but your nervous system, body memory, and energetic field. It's healing from the root, one cell at a time.

Divine Feminine
Not about gender, this refers to the sacred, intuitive, creative force within all of us. It's soft *and* fierce. Cyclical, embodied, and life-giving.

Dysregulation
A state where your nervous system is out of balance, often showing up as anxiety, shutdown, overwhelm, or hypervigilance. It's not weakness. It's a signal.

Embodiment
Living *in* your body, not just thinking about healing, but *feeling it, moving through it, and integrating it physically.* It's where your soul lands.

Integration

The sacred process of taking what you've learned or experienced and anchoring it into your body, choices, and lived reality.

Matrix

A term used in this book to describe the societal programming, systems, and illusions that keep us disconnected from our truth, power, and sovereignty.

Nervous System Regulation

Practices that help return your body to a state of safety, balance, and presence. This is foundational for healing, no amount of mindset work sticks without it.

Polyvagal Theory

A framework developed by Dr. Stephen Porges that explains how your nervous system responds to safety, threat, or shutdown. It helps decode your emotional and physiological states.

Rewilding

The act of shedding conditioning and returning to your natural rhythm, intuition, and power. A return to your wild, sacred self.

Sacred

Something deeply meaningful, spiritually connected, and rooted in reverence. In this book, "sacred" isn't religious, it's personal, embodied, and sovereign.

Sacred Rebellion

The act of returning to yourself in a world that taught you to abandon who you are. It's choosing alignment over approval, healing over hiding, truth over performance.

Somatic

Relating to the body. Somatic healing works through physical sensation, breath, movement, and body awareness to release trauma and reclaim wholeness.

Sovereignty

The remembrance that *you are your own authority*. That your body, your healing, and your choices belong to you. Not the system. Not the noise. You.

Printed in Dunstable, United Kingdom